W0010764

Ultimate Personal Power

Your Path to High Self-Esteem and Happiness

Laura Midna

Copyright © 2020 Laura Midna Inc. Publishing

Ultimate Personal Power: Your Path to High Self-Esteem and Happiness

All rights reserved. No part of this book may be reproduced in
any form without permission in writing from the author.

e-book: ISBN: 978-1-7772687-0-1
Paperback: 978-1-7772687-1-8
Hardcover: 978-1-7772687-3-2
Audiobook: 978-1-7772687-2-5

Formatting by Jen Henderson at Wild Words Formatting

DISCLAIMER

Neither the author nor the publisher of this work assumes any responsibility or liability of any kind on behalf of the consumer or reader and cannot be held responsible for the use of the information provided within this book. Always consult a trained professional before making any decision regarding treatment of yourself or others.

The resources in this book are provided for informational purposes only and should not be used to replace specialized training or professional advice of a healthcare or mental health professional.

Any perceived slight of any individual or entity is purely unintentional. Names and personal characteristics of the individuals have been changed to protect privacy. Events and timelines are distorted to protect privacy.

This book is not for everyone. It contains some adult themes. This book is intended for mature audiences. There are some trigger themes and words.

Feel free to reach out with questions:
lauramidna1969@gmail.com

Discover how to achieve high self-esteem and happiness today.
Tried and true practices with minimal time and money.
I learned from the best, and I am excited to share with you.

**Three percent of book profits will be given to the
Canadian Mental Health Association annually.**

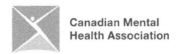

How important is happiness and high self-esteem to you?
What are you currently doing to address this?

I would like to dedicate this book to the following people:

The late Homer McDonald

He was the greatest mentor I could have imagined. His help gave me the tools I was looking for everywhere. I am forever humbled by his work with me.

My parents

They gave me everything they had.

Susie

An angel on Earth.

My precious children

I will love you for eternity.

G.A.

My love.

FOREWORD

If I were asked to describe this book in one word, I would call it Courage. For it takes rare courage to own your story and write it from your heart, which is exactly what Laura has offered in her book. It is a journey of discovery, from the depths of mental illness and struggles with self-esteem, to a place of stability and peace.

Renowned psychiatrist Bessel van der Kolk calls trauma and neglect the silent epidemic of our times, and this book, part memoir and part self-help manual, takes a very real look into the far-reaching impact of childhood neglect. One cannot help wonder how even well-meaning parents and caregivers can adversely affect the psyche of a developing child.

Yet, this book is a message of hope for people who have been through developmental trauma and neglect, and it illustrates how change is possible. Through years of therapy and self-help, Laura was able to overcome decades of mental illness and come to a place of personal power and identity. In this book, she shares some of the techniques through which she overcame her illness.

Volumes of psychiatric literature cannot compare to the lived experience of someone who has suffered from and overcome severe mental illness. Herein lies the power of this book. Not only is it a heart-wrenching honest look at the experience of mental illness, but more importantly, it offers hope that even the most severe illness can be overcome through persistent work on oneself. I hope it inspires everyone who reads it and instills hope that change is possible even in the most difficult of circumstances.

Dr. Dona Biswas
Author of *The Quantum Psychiatrist:*
From Zero to Zen Using Evidence-Based Solutions Beyond Medication and Therapy

CONTENTS

INTRODUCTION

....

The love which you give to yourself will be the most healing.

....

How does this sound? I would like you to tell a couple people you are reading a self-help book to help you stay accountable. John Corcoran, who was writing for the White House at twenty-three years old, and was pictured standing shoulder to shoulder with Presidents Bill Clinton and Barack Obama, said, "Trophies and ribbons do not go out to people who sit on the sidelines". We are going to take action. I am going to earn your respect, attention, and time. Tell your doubt and pessimism to sit down. We are going deep, but it isn't going to hurt. The ideas in this book are going to stretch you in a new direction. Parts may seem **polarizing** to you, but I guarantee the help portion will get you the goodies. For those with a severe mental illness history, this is going to have a big impact. For anyone else, this will be the vitamin you didn't know you needed. This is going to border on being fun. Everybody and their dog is offering self-help advice. Mine is different. Self-help with teeth.

As the song "Dirty Laundry" by Don Henley captures, there is a fascination with the ugly, but we all love a great success story. Through the case study of my life, I will show you the bottom of the mental illness barrel and how I reached a high level of self-esteem and happiness and how you can too.

There is no question in my mind that people who have been in the ring with mental illness are left with their self-esteem in shreds. I feel so strongly about the message in this book that I have left a directive in my will to ensure it crosses the finish line of publication, if something unforeseen happens to me. You will quickly see my life has been grey, so my thinking and approach to life is not black and white. **This book also has some lessons in diversity**.

If you were presented with tried and true practices for feeling great that were faster and more potent than traditional therapy and examining feelings, would it be worth committing to action? More gain, less pain? My goal is to *inspire* you, which is learning in its highest form. There is an emotional component to inspired learning. The information in this book is timeless and intended for anyone who believes we are stronger when we face reality eye to eye. Reality is the boss, and when we are equipped to deal with it and feel happiness and high self-esteem despite challenges, we are in a powerful position. This is not "I don't give a damn 1000 mg" but better. I want to give you value, and I am *driven* to share this information because it has turned my life around. You will not be able to *unsee* this information, and that is good news for your self-esteem and happiness goals.

Many people suffer with the pain of low self-esteem and diminished happiness. Often this is the result of happiness/success anxiety, self-criticism, worry, guilt, and feelings of inferiority/shame. This bleeds into all aspects of life. It has far reaching consequences to health, relationships, work, and the examples we set for our children. Our close circles get burned out trying to support us. When we whine, some people come to our rescue, but after a while, they get tired of it and want to stay away. Romantic love suffers because we burden our partner to make us happy and supply our sense of worth. It is a turnoff when people speak poorly of themselves, because it attacks pride—theirs and ours.

These issues affect normal people and are often amplified for those with serious mental illness history. People need to understand mental illness does not have the last word on your self-esteem and happiness. Overidentifying with being a victim keeps people trapped and helpless.

If I could download my experience and knowledge into your mind, I would. Since that is not an option, I have to trust my written word to reach you... to find, ignite your imagination, appeal to your sense of reason and engage your hope. Whether you are a garden variety sufferer or have a severe mental illness history, I am going to give you answers and insights. I will provide exercises to clear the path for happiness and high self-esteem. There will be some simple practices for handling items that come up every day and a formula for handling mistakes. I will also tell you how you can do something that protects and nurtures your romantic relationship. Happiness is nature's reward for successful action. This action will occur in the way you think, your behavior, and self-talk. I am here to tell you great things are in store for you. I am up at night with excitement thinking of how to inspire you to take action and stand by for your results. If you don't take control of your focus, the noise of conventional thinking and popular opinion will do it for you. *You have to get very clear about **wanting** high self-esteem and happiness.* There is no other way.

I have more mental illness experience than most people could shake a stick at. Since high school, I have been interested in psychology and human behavior. Desmond Morris' *The Human Zoo* and *Manwatching* were my favourite reads. I entered nursing as a graduate from a degree program and quickly gravitated toward psychiatric nursing. My career was in chronic and acute 'mental health'. I worked in the community with a crisis after-hours mobile mental health team. For many years, I worked in a community facility. I also worked in the hospital on an inpatient unit and, occasionally, an addictions floor. Over my life, I spent thousands of dollars on counseling from experts. I know what works. For a timeline perspective, I have searched for answers since the Berlin Wall came down. I am not selling novelty items like 'gamer girl bath water', which has gained importance these days! I am teaching life-changing information. My 31-plus years experience with numerous psychiatric problems, working in the field, and dedication to finding answers is at your fingertips. I've already done the heavy lifting. This is going to be a quick win for you.

Do you **want** the reality of high self-esteem and happiness? If you supply the *want,* I will supply the *methods.* I can show you an accelerated path. It is much closer than you think. Happiness is life-supporting. You will be more orientated toward finding humour, unlikely to burden others to help you feel good, and you will set a good example for your children. ***Your self-esteem will be a brick house instead of a straw one.*** You will not find self-esteem in a pill. Thankfully, the ideas don't have to be practised perfectly, so there is no pressure. Once you have insight, it will be easy to catch yourself in old patterns.

My biggest proof is myself. Today, I set limits with a client who looks for feelings of power by blatantly disrespecting women. I literally had cold chills from the strength of my boundaries immediately afterward. It was not always that way for me. I've been in the ring with mental illness for most of my life. I have suffered very much over the years, but now I identify strongly with people who have high self-esteem. I am happy and ready to face any challenge. I have a sense of control and a sense of humour. Objectively, most people treat me with more respect. We communicate our level of self-worth to others and they reflexively respond. I am not looking for others to fill holes in myself left from self-criticism and low self-esteem. My children get to experience a happy mom, not a mom who is worried all the time. They also get to see what high self-esteem looks like and therefore have a model to see it as normal for themselves.

To borrow a term from the gaming community, we want to stop *taking damage* from mental illness shame, and shame in general. Would it be good to push back against mental illness stigma?

In approaching the self-help portion of this book, I would like you to do so in the spirit of playfulness. If we look at the primary way in which children learn, we quickly see it is through play. This is evolution's answer to high demands for learning. If nature favors playfulness to assist learning in children, we can be sure it will benefit adults, as well.

Another lesson from children is a tolerance for setbacks. When a child falls while learning to walk, they don't quit and think, 'Walking is only for others'.

If you want to read the case study of my life, start at Part 1: One-stop shopping in the mental illness store. If you want to go straight to the self-help section, advance to Part 2: How to clean up from your shopping experience. Your choice. Your time. (In my head, I think that Part 1 is the qualifying round, with a hint of humor). When I want my teenage son to listen to wisdom, I ask him to "unlock" his brain temporarily. I would ask the same of you. One of the greatest unlocking tools for growth are the words "what if?" I am your biggest fan on this journey.

PART 1

1. My Early Years— Setting the Stage

I was an only child growing up. I had an adopted sister, Vanessa, who died of acute spinal meningitis at age seven before I was born. My mom loved Vanessa with all her heart. I believe a part of my mom died when Vanessa died. Mom was not able to eat, was fainting, and was hospitalized. She had to have another person look after me for months after I was born.

I think my mother was pretty much perfect at everything she did, although she was human with human flaws and vulnerabilities. She was beautiful, ambitious, witty, and outgoing. Her sense of humor left others with a feeling of value for having spent time in her company. She was so sharp, it was possible for her to disarm people in any way she chose— confrontation or humor. Sadly, she had grown up in an abusive home. Her arrival was unplanned, and her mother had nothing left to give. She witnessed her father chasing her mother with a knife, often. As a child, she concluded money would make her happy, so she had enormous anxiety around it all her life. She would say things like, "There is ten minutes of heat left in the oven after it is turned off," or "A fool and his money are soon parted". As a mother, she was a typical type A personality and was controlling. She was a victim of her own childhood, and was doing the best she could within her ability. In those days there was no "help" as we know it today.

Control is an interesting character trait because it gives one the sense of mastery in an unpredictable world. If a person can control their environment, and everyone in it, things feel safe and manageable. The need to control comes from people who are needy and perfectionistic. They lead a life script that tells them they need people and things to be a certain way to be happy. We have all come in contact with this.

My dad lived a long life. He had robbed the cradle by eighteen years in winning my mom. His personality was opposite to hers. He was quiet and steady. While courting, if she wanted his car with overdrive to go out with her friends, he was happy to give it to her. He was always generous. Once, he took her fishing and the current captured her. She panicked histrionically. Dad fished her out in a completely relaxed manner. Dad was genuinely benevolent and kind. Not as sharp as my mom, he compensated with a tireless work ethic. He was not a worrier, and I will tell you one of the ways that worked for him later in the book. Mom told me that Dad's best friend once said to him, "Alfred, don't you care about anything?" He was also a war veteran.

He gave me a great appreciation of nature and helped me catch minnows and tadpoles. I would eagerly await the spring sound of peepers in the pond signifying it was soon time to go collect frog eggs. He loved nature and kept me up to speed on the local wildlife. My dad always seemed more like a side character in our family, but he was setting a good example by being calm and patient. Mom called him dumb-smart. She often gave people nicknames.

And then there was me, a sensitive child who had a mother who loved her but was strict, a bit remote, and not affectionate. I was very obedient when I was a young child. I would not stand up for myself. I felt protective of my dad and would stand up for him when Mom was giving him a hard time. I was always artistically or creatively on fire over something.

I believe I internalized a lot of the anxiety my mom modeled. I developed asthma and had frequent headaches. I spent my time engrossed in art and the outdoors. Looking back, I can see that I began my studies of my mind very young. I used to pretend I was a horse motivated to trot to get chocolate-covered raisins. I also remember doing a type of meditation to improve my results on a test. Somehow, that information had filtered into my conscious awareness, but I cannot recall the source. My mom and dad always provided healthy food, and I loved to eat, but treats were in short supply. When I would visit friends' homes, I was always very interested in the treats. I also used to bum treats from kids at school. Food was a way to self-soothe.

The first event that showed me my mom's temper was around using the toilet. I would sit on the toilet to void, and urine would go between the seat and the bowl, running down the side of the toilet. At that time, we had a carpeted bathroom. It stands to reason that over a period of time it started smelling. I would try to fix the problem myself by repositioning myself on the toilet, but it wasn't working.

One day my mom, who was very house proud and extremely clean, discovered the problem and rubbed my nose in the carpet. My dad, who was very quiet and not confrontational, happened to come in at the same time. He addressed her by name and told her that was enough. This was the only time I ever knew him to stand up to her and speak with authority.

I doubled my efforts at repositioning myself on the toilet and also started using toilet paper as a dam to stop the problem for a couple years. It took me many years to figure out what was going on at that time, but I now believe my inner labia was directing the stream of urine in a horizontal position causing it to go between the seat and bowl. I was motivated to correct the problem without it being an issue for my mom, but since she had found out, it was increased pressure. Another incident when she lost control was over me losing a secondhand hat. It wasn't quite as intense, but both of these were surrounding the 'waste of money' by not taking care of property.

My asthma was an issue for my mom because she was so afraid I was going to die having already lost Vanessa. My episodes would intensify at night, and she would be up almost all night with me. She would be furious with my dad because he slept through it, night after night. She could not understand how he was not worried, especially because they had already lost one daughter.

I will never forget the look on her face as she watched me at night and sat up with me. It was an unhappy and deeply worried expression. I was finally taken to a specialist in a city and prescribed Intal, which was a theophylline drug used to treat asthma in those days. The specialist told Mom she should try to help me avoid intense emotions. I felt like I was not allowed to be too happy or angry at all. I was not allowed to watch "exciting" TV shows like the Bionic Woman or read Archie comics for this reason.

Trying to prevent a child from feeling the normal range of emotions seems like it would cripple emotional development. I remember when I was extremely happy about some relatives coming to visit, my dad told me to stop "showing off." I was allowed mild emotions but nothing intense. My asthma went into remission when I was about ten years old.

I know my mom loved me, but I didn't feel a connection with her. I self-comforted with food and thumb sucking for an extended time. I think it was the lack of physical affection that I was missing, but on some level, I feel I rejected her. She even said that to me at different times. She said I would close the door and say, "Most of all I like being lonely." I suspect I didn't trust her to be warm and nurturing, but I was also creative, so finding interesting activities was not difficult. Classical music was played in the home, and I remember one of my mom's favorite pieces was the Elizabethan Serenade. When I hear it now, it makes me think of 'feminine energy' and being 'light on one's feet'.

I was a bit of a misfit early on in school. I did have friends, but I was not embraced by peer groups. Starting in grade two, I had trouble grasping the work. By grade three, the school work was over my head, and I retreated into drawing on all my schoolwork. My report card reflected my difficulty, and I remember I had seven "needs improvement" scores. My mother hit the roof. She had me very scared. I called my best friend crying and saying I was scared. My friends were also scared of Mom.

I remember bringing my signed report card to my teacher the next day and the teacher said to me, "I pity you." I wasn't sure what she meant, but for years I thought she meant I was pathetic. My marks improved, but I remember it was very hard. By grade six, I was cheating on tests. I just couldn't seem to grasp math in particular. I am sure I had a learning disability, but those were not often diagnosed back in those days.

I started dissociating around this time when Mom would get very angry. Dissociation was involuntary for me, and it scared me in its own right. I felt like I was in a dream and I couldn't command my attention. I tried to explain it to my mom because it frightened me, but she didn't seem to understand. I also didn't want to go home after school.

There were funny things at this time, too, and usually around my mom's social life. My mom's best friend had a sister who was remotely an RN and more recently an attractive airline stewardess. Sometimes, she seemed to miss some obvious things and could be testy in nature. Once, my mom went to get some Jell-O from the fridge that Mary had made. It was not set, so my mom asked Mary how she had made it. Mom learned that Mary had measured a cup of boiling water and a cup of cold water. Then, entirely missing a step, she mixed the boiling water with the cold water before adding the Jell-O powder.

Another time there was a mix up with an answering machine. Mary answered a call from my mom but not before the answering machine started and Mary challenged "who were all these people on the phone?"

It was obvious to Mom and her best friend that Mary's dentist boyfriend was gay and had a boyfriend. They had been in a relationship for over twenty years and Mary was not tracking this.

In elementary school, I can remember being afraid of this girl who was older. She spit on a stick and made me put it in my mouth. I never told anyone, but I was intimidated by her. I was so submissive that I would never think of fighting back. I wish I would have punched her in the face. I also remember a schoolmate who had disfiguring burn scars on his face. He had lit a match to see inside a lawn mower gas tank. I was never afraid of him and never made a big deal about it like the other kids did.

My first trip away from home was with my cousin, Shelly. I visited her home, a six hour drive away from my hometown, for a few days. She was my appointed godmother. She was married and had children. My second cousins were close in age to me. I experienced her as warm, and she seemed happy. I felt free in a way I had not felt at home. I longed to live with her because it just felt good there.

When I was in grade five, I had a pony, after many years of obsession over horses. I drew endless horse pictures and talked about horses all the time. My mom was very indulging when it came to giving me opportunities. My mom nurtured me by spending money on me, but there were always undercurrents of anxiety and constant reminders around the need to be frugal and take care of things. Everything my mom touched was executed in a precise way. Horsemanship was no different. It was all done properly with a ferrier that came to our property, riding lessons, clinics, rallies, etc. My pony was difficult to control, and I was terrified of it, as well as my riding instructor, and I still didn't know my right hand from my left hand.

I was gratified with any pet I wished for, including guinea pigs, cats, angora rabbits, hamsters, gerbils and two ducks that left to go back to their original home. I had piano lessons, skating lessons, and lapidary classes to give expression to my love of geology. Mom supported my interest in art and bought the best mediums for me to work with, but, in keeping with her money anxiety, I used paper that was discarded from my dad's work. She encouraged me to enter contests, if I wanted. She wanted to cultivate my interest in activities. Her goal was that I would have choices and freedom as a woman. I also believe she wanted me to support her pride.

Throughout my childhood, Dad would have as much fun as I did with such things as helping me catch minnows. We made our own nets. He would go upstream and hit the water with cattails to scare the minnows into my net. I made a big production of the pollywog and minnow catching season. I had buckets upon buckets of frog eggs at various levels of emerging tadpoles. I was busy changing water and sorting them and releasing them when it occurred to me to be the right time. Dad had dug a sizable skating pond and it felt like a big deal to release minnows into that unstocked pond. I was impressed and amazed the minnows survived well and reproduced. I even imagined they had evolved some since the original ones we released. The minnows were hardy; they survived the pond nearly drying up and bounced back in good numbers. They used to sun themselves in the shallows of the pond when there was plenty of water.

We used to watch a lot of nature shows like Wild Kingdom and Science Magazine with David Suzuki. Much to my delight, Dad once caught me a little brown-nosed bat, which we released. We would take walks around the property and talk about the change of season and watch for new growth. He was a hunter and showed me how to fire a rifle, how to dress game, and took me saltwater fishing. When I was involved in Pony Club, he invested time daily toward stable management and pasture maintenance. Once, Mom told him to build me a treehouse. He built it two feet off the ground, but it was well done. This was the type of thing that Mom would roll her eyes at and he was told to smarten up and do it over. Dad used to like gardening, but mom did not favor his approach. She said, "Can't we have quality over quantity?" She tried to downsize his garden only to later discover "sneak gardens" in other places when she was out walking. Mom used to threaten my dad with getting a garbage man if he didn't stop salvaging things she would put in the garbage to be burned.

I used to ride every day. We had waterfront property and there was an elderly man who used to comb the vast marsh daily with a wheelbarrow instead of a shopping cart searching for something of value. In an oceanic setting, instead of the street, he was coordinating his searches with the tides. When I was out riding I would stop and he liked to tell me stories. He was always describing the same theme...stories of someone out to get him. His differentness did not frighten me in the least. Looking back I would say he was a paranoid schizophrenic. I don't think he thought it strange that a warm audience was arriving on horseback.

As I grew older, I became interested in showering and my appearance. If there was anything I desired most, it was to be beautiful. I had greasy hair at that age because of wearing a helmet for riding. I also had started having discharge. I wanted to change my underwear daily and wash my hair daily, but I was not allowed. I am pretty sure Mom's reason was that she did not want me sexually maturing.

I was bullied by one girl in my classroom because of my hair being greasy. My dad got up with me on school mornings, and he was fairly easy to sneak around. I started washing my hair in the sink downstairs. I also started planning to run away. I remember thinking that I could live on the school property in the woods and shower at the school gym and eat crackers. A friend called me "eccentric", and I think, if we are indexing people for words, "eclectic" is a softer word. Haha. Around that time, and in keeping with that word, I wanted to try eating frog legs. When unable to source them in the market, I fished/hunted my own. I will say I was always concerned about doing things in a humane fashion, as I learned from my dad.

I had a teacher who was a geologist, so the lab was 'decorated' with rock and mineral specimens. His love of geology spilled over into as much class content as he could get away with. This spilled right into me. I happily studied the Mohs Hardness Scale, used it, and liked the fingernail and glass references for perspective. I soon joined the geology club and became president. We went on a field trip to a place that had amethyst and found some pale pieces. My teacher identified a place to find garnet in shale, and Dad and I went off and found some good samples. I had some money one summer, and I found an amethyst geode which would take it all.

In those days, something that made me happy beyond measure was when we went to a cottage in the summer. It was near the ocean, and the beach was beautiful. I spent endless hours walking around and amusing myself. There were some interesting people in that community of seventy cottages, and Mom used to call them "storybook people". The cottage my parents bought was previously owned by some "pirate people". They used to fly the Jolly Rogers flag whenever my best friend Angelina's family was at their cottage. The pirate couple drank and smoked a lot, manicured their lawn with scissors, and would call the cops over rogue grass clippings. I knew there were artsy people in the community and I felt at home. I can remember the playground swings, the beauty, the warm water, sand in my bed, and fireflies. Looking back, these were the happiest times for my mom and dad too. My mom seemed more happy there and relaxed, and I am sure that contributed to my experience of being happy.

2. The Evolution of Problems

Becoming a pre-teen at this point, I will illustrate the power of suggestion to vulnerable girls around eating disorders. I was developing breasts very fast, and I had a strong desire to be beautiful. My mom had modeled control for me very well, and I was about to start using it. My self-esteem was very low.

I went with my mom to a friend's house. In a type of secrecy, my friend gave me a book. It was a book about a girl with anorexia nervosa and bulimia, and her name was Kesa. I devoured the book and started a diet. My mother was unaware of the book that was teaching me about bulimia. She seemed impressed by my initial efforts to lose weight, because she admired my commitment to a goal and not being overweight, which I was not. In a short period of time, I was addicted to the power of control I had with regard to my weight. This was something I could do well. It is always easy to connect the dots looking backward, and my need to be good at something had found expression.

I started becoming very restrictive, and then Mom became concerned. She started packing my favourite foods for lunch, but I was stronger than that for a time. As I had mentioned, I absolutely loved food, and it was one of the ways I nurtured myself. Resisting favourite foods became too difficult. I soon started purging after eating forbidden food, and that behaviour became dominant.

At this point, I had an attractive face and body, and my breasts were not too large. I was attracting the attention of boys, and some of that I liked. I attracted the attention of a black school mate and, although I wasn't interested in him, my mother found out. She said I must have been leading him on in some way. She was racist, and she hit the roof at a level I had not seen since grade three. She slapped my face, and I got a nosebleed. When I was a child, she was humored by me calling black people suntan people.

I took off for a ride on my pony and reported my mom to a friend's mom. There was a lot of conflict between Mom and me at this point, and I wanted to be away from home. My mom realized she had lost her cool and didn't want me to go to school the next day. I told her I was fine and would not tell anyone.

The next day at school, I talked to the guidance counselor and was taken from the home. I can't imagine what that was like for my mom, but I know it started a rift in my relationship with my dad that was never repaired.

I lived away with a family for a few months and then returned home with some conditions. I previously had not been allowed to decorate my room at all, and I wanted to be able to personalize it. I also had a new lock on my bedroom door, which was short lived but unnecessary in the first place.

It was around this time that I started smoking with the bad kids. I was very hostile toward my mom and hell-bent about doing what I wanted to. Other kids my age were permitted to hang out at the mall and I was not. I was also not allowed to go to school dances. I started leaving the house and hitchhiking if I wanted to go somewhere.

I understand, in retrospect, that my mother felt I was not making good choices, but I felt hard done by and was angry. I had started cutting my arm by this point with knives. I would cut mostly with intense emotions like jealousy and anger. In fact, one time while my mother was yelling at me, I cut the back of my hand with a comb. I lacked any skills to deal with intense emotions. Sometimes when I was angry I would write. My mother would call these "pencil fits". My eating disorder was my comfort, and oddly it served both of us, as it kept me in step with my mother's fear of me maturing sexually.

I was well liked by the less popular kids in the school and also had some popular friends around this time. There were some very funny people in my class, and I had my mom's great sense of humour so I spent a lot of time laughing. I would stay indoors at recess to be in the company of a schoolmate who would nearly have me on the floor with laughter.

He was definitely the eccentric type. He was also an artist with an obvious crush on me, and he drew an impressive portrait of me from a photograph.

I won the winter carnival queen contest that year in grade nine. I was accused of asking the nerds to vote for me. My mom thought it went to my head. She said attractive girls are a dime a dozen. I also was bullied by a very scary girl because I was not interested in her friend who still liked me. This was the same guy my mother lost her mind over. She said I thought I was the beautiful bitch and said I was racist. I was terrified of her. I knew full well she could beat the crap out of me, and I was still not the type to fight back. She was tough as nails and was older than me. Many years later, I heard she had become a prostitute.

We had neighbours at this point who had some bad boy teenagers, and I had my first full fledged crush. Needless to say, I was not allowed to date Rick, so I would sneak around to see him and was absolutely infatuated with him. I can still remember the smell of his leather jacket and cigarettes. Rick often went to the arcade, which was another place I was not allowed to go to.

3. Private School Away From Home

My mother was desperate to keep me away from "riff raff," as she called them. She approached me that summer about going to a private school. I was motivated to be away from her and have more freedom, so that seemed like a great offer.

Before I went away to school, I had a summer job at a fast food joint that sold ice cream. I was able to manage serving ice cream, but the more prestigious work was cooking at the grill. This was my first confirmation in the real world that I was not organized, and it was recognized by my boss. It was not that I was unmotivated, but my boss could see I was below average in my abilities. It was never discussed, but the fact that I was never assigned to the grill validated my suspicion that I was less. The only person who believed in me was my mom, and it was blindness. Reality always has the last word.

Private school was great for me socially. I had more freedom there, but I was still struggling very much academically. There was always plenty to laugh about. The cafeteria was a great thing for a person with bulimia because there was no end to the amount of food I could eat. I was having a hard time with my self-esteem, however, because my breasts had grown very large, and the slender look was still very much in fashion. I also hated my nose. I would sit in class with my hand shielding my nose.

Smoking continued to be a comfort for me. My asthma stayed in remission. The trick was being able to smoke without being busted by the prefects. Prefects were the same as student police who had a limited amount of power to oversee student behaviors and handle them accordingly or report to the duty teacher, headmistress, or headmaster in serious instances. I was not yet sixteen and did not have my parent's permission to smoke. Around the time of my 16th birthday, I forged my mom's signature and gave myself permission to smoke without involving my parents at all.

There was a biology teacher who seemed to understand that I had some academic difficulty but was very interested in biology. I did extremely well one year but failed the genetics part miserably because of the math component. I had hoped my enthusiasm would win me the biology award that year. The girl who took the award aced everything. The teacher acknowledged me by offering me a reading opportunity. He presented me with the book *The Human Zoo* by Desmond Morris, and I absolutely loved it. I also gained acceptance with another teacher who didn't make me feel less for my inability to grasp math. He has remained a lifelong friend, a friend of my differentness. He is a great person with a good sense of humor and has supported me as a person all these years.

I had a love interest at this time even though he did not compare to Rick, whom I was still writing letters to. He wasn't everything I was looking for, but I wanted to go all the way with him.

Being that it was a coed private school, there were separate boys and girls dorms, but they were connected. I knew the penalty for sneaking into the boy's dorm would be expulsion. Similar to the girls' dorm, there were teachers who patrolled the dorms at regular intervals during the night.

I was determined, so I snuck up to my boyfriend's room that he shared with another boy. It was thrilling for the time it lasted. I didn't get caught and made it back to my room. I had been planning on becoming sexually active for a while, so I was on the pill. Free samples were available from the school nurse, and I had taken no chances as I knew my mom would have lost her mind.

The next morning when I was going to class, my knees felt weak and rubbery. It was a remarkable sensation and the first, and only, time I had ever felt it in my life. The unexpected part was feeling suicidal the following night. I had a sneaking suspicion that my boyfriend was bi-sexual, and, at that time, I felt that meant something shameful. I felt like the shame was on me for sharing that special first time with someone who I didn't feel measured up in my mind. It made me feel bad about myself and made me feel more worthless.

4. SUICIDE ATTEMPT

That evening, I took an overdose of allergy pills and analgesics. (What I would like you to know, if you support a youth who has suicidal ideation, is that an attempt can be very impulsive.) It was just before supper when I took the overdose. In retrospect, I know I intended it to be high lethality.

By the time I went to the sit-down meal, I was somewhat high. We had prefects at every table, and I was sitting close to one. He asked me what was going on with my breathing. I had not realized anything was happening with my breathing. I said there was "nothing wrong."

After supper, I figured I had not taken enough medication, so I took more. I had a brief few moments of wanting help and went to see the school nurse and made a weak display that something was wrong, but she was busy and did not pick up on my bid for help. I went back to my room.

There was a very beautiful girl who used to come to me for massages. I wanted to look like her so badly. I thought if I was attractive enough, I would like myself. She had a wicked personality, full of confidence. She was a little bit androgynous. I wanted to be her friend, but she mostly used me. She dabbled in drugs and picked up on something not being right with me. She kept asking me what I was on because she wanted some. I kept denying there was anything, but I know she didn't believe me.

I went to bed at the lights out time and was hallucinating that my bed sheets were a newspaper. I believed I would never wake up again. I awoke sometime during the night and had a hallucination that my roommate was a cross between my mother and the physics teacher, who had a similar temperament as my mom when he was angry. He instructed me to go to the bathroom, and I was sick throwing up coffee grounds-like matter. I was also hallucinating that there were colourful fish in the toilet.

After that, I went back to bed and knew that I would probably be waking up in the morning. I did wake up, and I started the day in the usual way but felt very depressed. A few days later, I made a less serious suicidal attempt by spraying about half a cup of Raid bug killer into a glass and drinking it. The only thing that happened with that was terrible chemical burps.

I went through the motions of living and carried on until my grade twelve year. I was completely overwhelmed with the difficulty of the curriculum, and I failed grade twelve. I hated my body so much, and to make matters worse, the sergeant major at my school, where we had mandatory cadets, was exploiting my need for cigarettes with the effect of making me feel shame. We seemed to have a trade going on where I could smoke his cigarettes in his office and he got to talk to me about my breasts and draw pictures of what he thought they looked like. He asked me to show him where my nipples were situated on the drawings. I feel that he was baiting me to show him my breasts. It made me feel shameful because I was always trying to hide my large breasts, but the need for cigarettes was stronger.

I remember a specific incident that further compounded my shame of my breasts. A boyfriend I had a relationship with in grade twelve planned an overnight trip away with me during the Chinese New Year celebration week. We had not been intimate up until then. When I disrobed and approached him while he was sitting on the bed, he kicked me away from him. The experience was humiliating. It was difficult to process some of these things.

There was also another incident where I had gone to the classroom building in the evening to try and do computer work. The building was not staffed and there were only a very few of us there. When I left the computer lab, I was followed and pinned down on the stairs. The fellow student wanted me to suck him off. I thought quickly and said there was someone coming and he let me up.

I reported him to the headmaster the next day, and the headmaster's response was for me to stay away from him. I think that was not a great response in a school where my parents were paying tuition. I carried on and stayed the hell away from him. The days continued to unfold, and I gave some thought to what I would do after school.

I had decided I wanted to be a nurse with my mother's encouragement, but I had to repeat grade twelve. It was hard to be left behind repeating a school year, but I applied myself and was motivated to try my best with my mother in the background. My mother was correct in that she wanted me to have options and not need a man for financial security. She saw education as a means to this end. I had a desire to help people, but I certainly was not equipped. My mother told me to read a book called *Nurse Heal Thyself First*. I didn't read it and resented the perception of my mother putting me down. I knew I had problems, but I had zero insight about what could help and thought my mother was to blame. I knew that book was going to underdeliver, at least in my case.

5. Attempts at Normalcy

Before I entered university for the Bachelor of Science in Nursing program, I finally had a chance to have sex with Rick. I still thought he was incredible. Once in university, I was minimally focused on work as soon as I discovered how difficult it was. I had a boyfriend, for a period, who was gifted in intelligence. I marvelled over his mind. He effortlessly tutored me in a research statistical course I would have otherwise failed. I concentrated on smoking, eating, hanging with friends, and going to bed with fellas in search of self-esteem. I understand it was misguided and wrong.

There was a girl in my nursing class who was drop-dead gorgeous. She was also sweet and became a good friend. More than anything, I wished I could have looked like her. I imagined how perfect her life was because she was beautiful. I was always in awe of beauty, beautiful color arrangements, jewelry, furniture, or abandoned houses and all their beauty and history. I would take any opportunity to get inside one. I found a couple with old glass doorknobs and imagined I would someday have glass doorknobs in my home. I even went into the attic of my grandfather's house looking for old artifacts.

In university, there were two fellas who really stood out in my mind because of their self-assurance. The first was studying fine arts and was very good looking. He was extremely confident, and he had his eye on me at a party. His vibe was bigger than Billy be damned. I felt him staring at me, and all he had to do was come over and pick me up and carry me upstairs and have his way. He kept contact with me afterward, and I really wanted a relationship with him. He lost interest in me over another female who was not especially attractive, but she had solid self-esteem.

The second fella was a black man from the Bahamas. He was visiting friends at the university. He had that same confident vibe and without any hesitation sat me on his knee. It took me a long time to get both of these men out of my mind.

My other focus was food. There was an all-you-can-eat scenario in the cafeteria. Usually, I would eat until I could not eat another thing and go to a bathroom and purge and then go back a second time to do the same thing. I figured I could eat about three quarts of food. I was bingeing and purging as many as eight times a day. It was to the point that I didn't know when to take my birth control pill because I was afraid it wouldn't be absorbed. I knew how to layer the food in my stomach for the easiest and most complete purge. I also had to be careful about selecting bathrooms for discretion and fast access to reduce the amount of calories absorbed. I had sores and calluses on my knuckles from my teeth.

I did realize my eating disorder was out of control, and I tried to seek help with my nutrition professor "asking for a friend." My professor seemed confused and not willing to help. I booked an appointment with mental health services at the hospital. The appointment is worth mentioning.

For intake purposes, I was interviewed and I was asked some questions from the mini mental exam and the GAF (Global Assessment of Functioning). It is a standardized assessment tool to determine functioning and cognitive impairment. When I was asked to do some basic math computations, I felt immediately defective and literally ran out of the office. My eating disorder was certainly out of control. I experienced palpitations daily from my disturbed fluid balance. Excessive vomiting depletes potassium, which is necessary, particularly, in heart function.

The degree nursing program was quite new in those years, and I knew I was pushed through more than on my own merit. Remarkably, I passed the RN exam. Although I was never sorry I had a university education, I now understand, as a parent, the danger in pushing a youth against their grain.

My mom wanted me to be successful and have a better life. She wanted me to aspire to be a nurse manager. I did not have the aptitude for that, and I am careful not to push my children against the grain as I realize it imposes unnecessary stress and wastes time. Let what is natural flow from a person.

I had my mind set on getting away from a winter climate, so when a nurse recruiter came to the university and was offering jobs at a hospital in Houston, Texas, I was all for it.

Before my employment was due to begin, I had one last summer at home. It was interesting for me. I was waitressing and a couple things happened. The first thing dawned on me over the period of a couple days. One of the cooks in the kitchen was female but had more male traits. She was always nice to me, but it surprised me after a few shifts that I felt attracted to her. It was a bit exciting and added an extra element of enjoyment to my work. She was quite a bit older than me, and I don't know if she perceived my interest, but I wasn't about to act on it. It was merely a curiosity, and I was amused by it.

The second thing that happened was being approached by a mud wrestling troupe called the Chicago Knockers. They were visiting to perform locally. They wanted to recruit me. I was intrigued by that world, although I was only imagining what it might be like. I was flattered thinking they thought my face was pretty enough, but I hated my breasts, and I was determined that I was going to have breast reduction surgery sooner than later.

I believed, and still believe, that what is "natural" to humans is manipulation of looks if so desired. People changing their hair colour, shaving and makeup is a manipulation. I think if people want cosmetic surgery or implants or lip fillers or whatever, they should go for it. Madonna is off-the-hook beautiful these days. Other cultures alter their looks through patterned skin scarring, neck rings, historical foot binding and lip plates to name a few. Body adornment and manipulation, for the purpose of looks, is *natural* to humans and not unique to Western culture and it is not a new concept. Some people prefer a "natural" look and leave nature alone. It is individualized and sometimes culture driven.

My mother was unwilling to let me take the time for breast reduction surgery before I set off on my first job as a RN. My breasts were larger than DD34. I had stopped measuring and stuffed myself into that size bra. Mom called it "unnecessary surgery." I felt that she liked that my breasts held my confidence back and kept me more tame. I set my goal that once I was out on my own, it would be a priority. The first step was to find employment.

Although I knew my interest was in psychiatric nursing, I felt that a job in cardiovascular telemetry would round me out as a nurse. That was the job I had been offered. Well, I can tell you that my orientation was a nightmare. I knew I was not smart enough to work on the unit and would pose a risk to patients. The last thing I wanted to do was cause harm. I was crying every day before I went to work so I terminated my employment. My mother didn't talk to me for months. I was about twenty-two years old.

6. Mental Health As a Career

I moved away with my boyfriend, who was originally from the UK, and worked at a gas station, had my breast reduction surgery and rhinoplasty, and then found work in psychiatric nursing. That boyfriend was a good fella. He was supportive and patient. Comically, before we ever bought a car, we rented a car to go to a place in order to look for rocks. It was a wild goose chase, and there was some off-roading required. I was able to get to a rhodonite site with other rock collectors, where I found some samples. I also tried gold panning. My boyfriend shared my enthusiasm for cars and taught me to drive standard, which became a prerequisite in choosing cars, as well as a lifelong passion. He was mechanical, and that turned me on. Since initially becoming licensed to drive, I had a fixation with Corvettes and test drove many used ones when I could find them. I also had a great experience driving a 70-½ Camaro before learning standard. Loved that torque.

I was deeply interested in mental illness. More than anything, I wanted to gain insight into abnormal psychology, understand it, and make a difference. I somehow knew all behavior was goal-driven. I didn't want to be a cog in the wheel, and I had a suspicion that medication had its limits. Schizophrenia was very hard to understand, and I wondered a lot about the nature/nurture divide in its development. I had felt there was a strong nurture component, but I remember going to courses where they refuted that. I was dismissively given the message I didn't know what I was talking about. It was the '90s and nurses were minions in the psych community. The medical model was the only accepted framework for delivering care and treatment.

I decided to just keep observing and make a difference in small ways where I felt I could. I couldn't help but study the clients I worked with. Everyone had a story that was often hard to get to the bottom of because of the level of impairment caused by positive and negative symptoms, predominantly with chronic schizophrenia. Add to that, many clients were institutionalized. That means a person has become less independent in thinking and behaving as a result of living in a care facility for an extended period. Not all my clients had schizophrenia, but there was a high representation of it. I remember an elderly client who was so kind and so hard working I am at a loss for words to describe him other than to say he turned himself inside out to be of service to others. God bless him. He had so many reasons to feel a sense of pride, but I know he had none. If the embodiment of self-effacement could be defined by a person, he was the poster child. There are many clients I remember but I am just mentioning a few.

I worked with a client who I identified as a water intoxicant and nobody believed me. Without funds for drugs, he had discovered he could alter his consciousness and escape by drinking excessive amounts of water. I was finally believed when he had a seizure because of this behavior. It was me who found him while he was having a seizure, and he was incontinent of urine. I called 911, and he was taken to the hospital by ambulance. He was hospitalized, stabilized, and once discharged, his care plan reflected a new protocol. The new care plan was implemented with minimal success as we did not have physical control over his access to taps. He was at least monitored more closely and eventually moved to a different group home. One of my colleagues had known him in high school, and he was a partier, but otherwise normal until that critical period for males, in particular, just before adulthood.

I remember a client who I felt had never had a sincere compliment in his life. He was marginalized as a First Nations person. When I commended him on his great sense of humor and terrific memory, I felt how brittle he was. A serious, concerned anxiety came over him. Normally he was always joking and laughing. Other staff used to find him irritating, but I always thought he was very ill but still knew how to laugh and enjoy himself. I liked his personality. I know my clients felt visible to me, but I could offer little more than that at the time. I continued observing and questioning over the years.

There was a client who could be extremely violent and had organic aspects disposing him to mental illness. He had a dual diagnosis. His old chart notes from the asylum, which was downsizing, described that he had once excelled in mathematics. It was still possible to see deep intelligence. He had assaulted a staff member with a 50-pound rock. He wore a helmet because of seizures, but staff had no such protection. I was leery of him because he was big and, tragically, young. One morning, I was prompting him to make his bed. He completed the task and then, happily and without warning, picked me up to thank me in a bear hug that was terrifying. Another night after I finished my shift, I headed out to my car, which was parked on the street. He jumped out from behind my car and said "Boo" with child-like delight. He scared the shit out of me. I think I might have been a smaller target for his anger because he liked my personality, but I never let my guard down because he could be unpredictable.

When I had days off, I was having fun going to the local rock shop and finding expensive specimens and buying them and waiting for new ones to appear. Sadly the rock shop burned down. I brought my rock collection in to share with the clients in the group home. It made me happy and I thought they might enjoy the beauty. It was shortly after I heard I had been sarcastically named the queen of the facility by the manager. She must have resented my passion.

By the time I was 28, I was becoming bored with my boyfriend, which was my typical pattern. I had many boyfriends since my teens, and although I had been dumped occasionally, most of the time I was the one who became bored and left.

I later learned from the writings of Homer McDonald, B.S., M.Ed. that it was low self-esteem that caused me to get bored and leave. Once I felt I had the fella wrapped and he was no longer a challenge, my interest disappeared. Homer said that this is a subconscious process whereby at a deep level I did not think I was that great, so once I had the devotion of a fella, I looked down on him for being in love with me. So here again, I left that boyfriend. I did not expect what was coming next.

Almost immediately after my boyfriend left and returned to the UK, I started experiencing unmanageable anxiety. I was waking up in the morning with waves of panic. It was very hard to eat anything. I was sure I had mono or something of a physical nature.

My hands were sweating profusely, constantly. I had never had sweaty hands before in my life. I felt like if I talked my words would be garbled. It was absolutely terrifying and unrelenting.

I leaned heavily on my girlfriend and felt highly anxious to be without her. I could have upstaged a wet hen. I went to my doctor who diagnosed me with generalized anxiety disorder and prescribed antidepressants and anti-anxiety medication. I felt ashamed and defective and did not take the medication.

Working during those days was absolute torture. My anxiety became so great that I was dissociating at work and trying to hide how sick I was. It was so difficult because I was afraid to speak, I couldn't command my attention out of the dissociation, and I was terrified. I worked one on one with a lot of clients, and because they were so profoundly ill, they were not noticing. I was certain that I was going to become schizophrenic. One of my nurse friends laughed at me for saying that. I had myself on a very tight mental health leash. Something that I was very averse to was science fiction movies. I was fearful that any suspense of my disbelief would certainly send me into psychosis. My mom did not know the entire extent of my suffering, but suggested I take the seven-hour flight and move home. I insisted I couldn't move home until I fixed myself.

7. Spending a Lot of Money on Counseling

Interestingly, sometimes after my shifts, I had some relief from my symptoms. Other times I can remember going on punishing walks on steep inclined hills to try and make my anxiety go away. I hated it, and those walks never worked. I often had no appetite and had to drink Ensure to maintain food intake. I tried the program *Awaken the Giant Within* that my boyfriend owned. I liked it, but it did not help with the anxiety. I tried breath work with a facilitator and Reiki treatment. I also tried a tapping procedure and acupuncture. I was willing to submit myself to anything but medication to help. I treated it like an executive order and supplied a machine-like commitment. I even started entertaining thoughts of shock therapy, but never a frontal lobotomy. Obviously it was not an option but, unfortunately, probably never a choice for those who had it, in the past.

I started reading self-help books at a local coffee shop where I could smoke. The first book I read talked about acting "as if". I was motivated to try, so I went to work and acted as if I was confident. I was able to do it for about five minutes, and immediately noticed a completely different reaction from the staff I was speaking to. She responded as if I really was a confident person. I had never felt that before. I abandoned it, however, because I didn't think it could work if I didn't have the internals to support it. I found Nathaniel Branden's work on self-esteem and conceptually felt that everything he wrote was true. I was certainly getting an education on how I should conduct my life to have good self-esteem, but it was doing very little to help with the intense anxiety I was experiencing. I was also not feeling good self-esteem. I decided to try harder and took telephone sessions with Nathaniel and eventually went to California to have sessions with him in person.

Los Angeles, California was incredible to me. I stayed at a hostel around Hollywood and managed to see some points of interest. I couldn't believe Rodeo Drive. I was very interested in fine jewelry, anything beautiful. There was an estate jewelry store I went to. I was wearing a costume jewelry ring with a light pink stone in it. One of the jewelers said to me that he had an actual diamond the colour of my pink stone. He said he would have to ask permission to see if I could view it. He brought out a silk fabric cloth and unwrapped a loose pink diamond. The colour was very intense, and it blew my mind. I am estimating it was .25 carats. He even let me use my disposable camera to take a picture of the diamond with my finger next to it for perspective. I was very gracious of him taking the time and interest to show it to me, and I thanked him.

In Santa Monica, I was charmed into going to a strange man's house so he could work on my chakras hoping that would help. First, we went to a restaurant named Gladstones. We went in his older Maserati. I was fine until he wanted to access some chakra which required him to breathe air into me with his mouth on mine. I didn't know much about chakra treatment, but it sounded sus to me, so I said I wanted to leave. He didn't seem to want to drive me back, so I insisted he give me cash for a cab to get back to Hollywood. He did. My boyfriend at the time nearly lost his mind.

I actually went to the Beverly Hills Hotel for lunch. I was surprised they allowed me in. I ate my lunch by the poolside and had the most delicate miniature blueberry muffins with tea and a sterling teaspoon. I loved that experience.

On my appointment day, I was very star-struck to meet Nathaniel. He lived and practised from his home in Beverly Hills. He had been a friend to Alan Greenspan, and had a romantic history with Ayn Rand. (I had changed my name legally, inspired by Ayn's name change. I had picked a name which I thought would confer sexiness and self-love the name promised). I was so anxious about being on time for my appointment that I arrived twenty minutes too early, by taxi, at his residence. I was told I had arrived "far too early" as a reprimand.

At the time, I thought Nathaniel's work was incredible, and his writing was almost poetic. I did not have any sexual interest in him, but I was in awe of him. I had three sessions with him. I had sold my sports car and had bought a very old but mechanically sound tank of a car called a Dodge Omni to be able to afford the trip and counseling.

I remember one session where I was feeling dissociated and I was sitting on his butter yellow couch. I moved on the couch and noticed a dark stain on the couch that looked like a wet spot. I was scared I had left it and had to ask him immediately if I had done that. It would be atypical of my bodily functions, but I had not noticed it when I sat down and was questioning my ability to apprehend reality. Please appreciate that in a dissociated state, one feels disconnected from much of what is going on. He said, "No, unfortunately I had a client sitting there who had a bottle of shampoo in her purse and it leaked."

We worked on sentence stem exercises and hypnosis. After my sessions with him were complete, I had some things to work on in an effort to help myself. I continued on to San Diego to meet my first cousins for the first time. I was very excited to go but again felt dissociated for most of the visit. I was disappointed that Nathaniel had not been able to give me the magic bullet.

When I returned home, I continued telephone sessions with Nathaniel. I had it in my mind that I was not executing his advice well enough. I was always measuring myself against the requirements he had written about to achieve self-esteem. He had outlined everything in great clarity. During the first phone session, he asked me if I had gone out there looking to get into trouble sexually with him. He said that he felt I was trying to confirm my belief that men could not be trusted. I was surprised by that, but in light of the couch incident, I could see how he came to that conclusion. I just figured he really had no idea of my level of anxiety, dissociation, and distress. He did open my mind about happiness anxiety and reclaiming disowned parts of the self. I just arrived at high self-esteem in a different way.

8. PONDERING MENTAL ILLNESS

There was something in Nathaniel's book that was speaking to me. He had written "A flight from reality is often a flight from one's inner state" (Branden, 1994, p. 40). I think he intended it to mean escape, but not psychosis. Since I was still both afraid and curious about schizophrenia, it stuck with me.

I also was thinking that there was lots of evidence that said the onset of schizophrenia is at the threshold of adulthood. It is at this point that the supports fall out from the family and the individual is faced with using their life skills to be self-supporting. There is so much truth in the statement that the proper aim of parenthood is to provide roots to grow and wings to fly.

When I thought about my clients who had schizophrenia, most of them seemed impoverished in their life skills set aside from their symptoms. I am not about to argue that there is not a genetic predisposition for schizophrenia, but there seems to be a strong nurture component.

Sometimes abuse in childhood can result in the absence of learning life skills. This can occur by neglect or the youth is so preoccupied with the trauma that there is no opportunity for learning. Add to this, if a youth develops addictions, their emotional and life skills development gets arrested. Not as dangerous, but still harmful, is the parent who infantilizes their child by being over-protective with the result being the child does not learn self-sufficiency and confidence. As much as I could, I tried to help clients learn better life skills. It was a struggle with my own impairment, but I wanted to help. I had a client who could not tell time, and I know that he was not below average intelligence. He had described being forced to eat vomit as a child. With that type of abusive environment, it is not hard to imagine there was little room for normal developmental learning to occur.

Schizophrenia, which is a thought disorder, is typified by delusionals as a main symptom. It is interesting that a common theme in delusions is one of grandiosity. It fits that a person who experiences themselves so powerless experiences delusions where they have super powers and are god-like. I had arrived at this conclusion in my late 20s, long before I read *How to Win Friends and Influence People*. I was happy to read it in Carnegie's book, which I read in my 40s. I don't think the person with schizophrenia consciously experiences themselves as powerless since they are delusional, but somewhere inside them there is knowledge and probably all at a subconscious level. "Some authorities declare that people may actually go insane in order to find, in the dreamland of insanity, the feeling of importance that has been denied them in the harsh world of reality" (Carnegie, 1981, p. 22).

Could Carnegie be suggesting the need for self-esteem is so important that people go insane to find it? Yet the following seems true. I believe evolution pushes some differences in creativity within the gene pool to give us a species advantage. Somehow, nature already knows the price may be mental illness, so deviance is expressed in a few. Life always has an eye on the future and sees that experimentation has value. Just like us, natural selection also wants to peek around the corner and is almost playful.

When I looked at myself, I was starting to realize that my perfect mother had over-helped me in many ways. I allowed this because she was so capable and I had some degree of a learning disability. I was more than happy for her to do everything despite all the conflict. On the rare occasion when I appeared to like myself, my mom would knock me down by saying, "Don't we think we are wonderful?" I thought about it for years, but recently concluded it was a control maneuver.

Conflict also confers a dependency. People often think of dependency as a passive state, but this isn't always the case. If a person is truly emerging as an autonomous individual, they are not in conflict all the time with a parent or other person. They just do what needs to be done and consult others for perspective or objectivity.

Pondering Mental Illness

When I had ended the relationship with my boyfriend, I was alone as an adult, and I think I had the life skills of a fourteen year old. I had a smoking addiction, bulimia, poor self-esteem, and was in denial of my learning disability and lower than average intelligence. It would take many years before I could come to terms with those because my self-esteem was already so fragile. Stanton Peele wrote, "Addictions are difficult to ferret out of the individual because they fit the individual" (Peele, 1999, p.46). As an example, someone who has a food addiction is often seeking comfort, and someone who has a coke habit often wants to feel powerful. My addictions centered around the need to self-soothe and manage anxiety. Reading Peele's book was another attempt to gain some leverage over what was happening with me.

For timeline purposes, I was in my late twenties and dating a successful fella, but there were problems. I was learning how to ride a motorcycle and preparing to get licensed. I bought a Honda CBX 250. I was loving my time off going to Starbucks and drinking caramel frappuccinos, smoking, and reading. I loved tabloid magazines and fashion magazines. I was still consumed by a desire to be beautiful, not aware this was a need for self-esteem.

9. The Lure of More

As often as I could, I was going to the local strip club out of fascination and a belief that strippers might have the answer to self-esteem. Was it possible that the attitude of not giving a fuck was what I needed to achieve? I absolutely loved going, and wished I could be a stripper. The dancing, costumes, and music was napalm. The relationship I was in came to a head when I found my boyfriend was hiding liquor and pot. The tipping point was when he shook me by the shoulders over me going to the strip joint. He reached out to my mom and said he wanted to marry me but couldn't control me. I still had feelings for him, but I left and white-knuckled through the pain, channelling my energy into drawing a great picture of him. I used driving and music to settle my heart.

I read a couple books looking for relationship insights. One was *Why Men Love Bitches* by Sherry Argov. Then I read *The Rules* by Sherrie Schneider and Ellen Fein. The other book was *Loving Him without Losing You* by Carolyn Bushong. She was very results oriented and I had one telephone consultation with her. I read one book, and I can't remember which one for sure so I am not going to offer a best guess. The book suggested I needed to confront my parents for how they failed me in order to heal. I was set for a trip home so I prepared mentally to do this. It's suggestion meant I had to follow through with the recommendation although I was being ruthless in an attempt to heal myself. Confronting mom was nothing new but I had never confronted my father before and he did not deserve it. I still believed my troubles were entirely the result of my childhood. I confronted my benevolent dad saying he failed to protect me from my mom. He didn't say anything back but he couldn't command his speech for the next couple days which was concerning. Worse, we set out to take my kayak to the lighthouse and when he tried to load it I could recognize he was dissociated.

I was wearing a jacket and pants combination rain suit. I could have died twice that day. I was travelling alone for a distance of about twelve miles coming in with the tide in the channel where large ships passed in the highway between the red and green marker buoys. I was not thinking about my dad for the afternoon. For fun I approached the green buoy and found a way to anchor myself to it and enjoyed that perspective. I loved being out in my kayak close to the water with the opportunity to see large vessels. The experience of being so close to the water and exploration of the ocean was incredibly interesting to me. (One other time in a local lake I had rescued a duckling that was caught in a fishing line).

Once I reached the inner harbour I paddled up beside a very large docked ferry. It transported people, 18 wheelers and many passenger vehicles. I liked being close to it for the difference in size. I could see from many small whirlpools that the stern thrusters were on. A man came out and told me promptly to get out of there because there was undertow and I could be pulled under. I immediately realized the danger and paddled away as fast as I could. I was feeling lucky he was there to see the danger for me and had likely saved my life. I paddled on to the spot where my dad would meet me to remove the kayak. He was able to see where I was by using binoculars. He coordinated the time perfectly. As I was getting out I realized an oversight. The yellow rain gear had caused me to forget my lifejacket. I never said a word to my dad about either and I don't believe he noticed. I was thankful I only noticed at the shore because had I made the discovery while essentially out at sea I would have panicked. Dad was still shaken as he drove the wrong way on a familiar one way street. It was tragic to hurt him in this way.

Time rolled on, and in 1999 I learned that I had some precancerous cells on my cervix, so I decided to stop taking my birth control pill. I felt my biological clock was ticking. I did not want to be a parent, but I wanted to have a child. I explored getting inseminated with a man's semen in a situation where his wife was not conceiving. It was a type of surrogacy arrangement. The agreement was I would give the baby to them, and I knew they would be incredible parents. I had known them both for a few years. We undertook the challenge with a turkey baster, although I know they would have welcomed me into their bedroom. I was not successful in conceiving.

I met a fella who I was not initially attracted to, but he seemed kind to me and was persistent. I grew to be attracted to him, and we had a relationship for a time. He was happy to go along with my stripper interests, and we went to the club all the time. I got to the point of entering two amateur contests. My boyfriend said I was "mechanical" in my performance, and I did not pursue it further. I rather enjoy dancing!

I remember one night we went to a stripper club and there was a blond who had thick thighs and cellulite. She had a gorgeous face, and her costume was beyond beautiful. I will never forget her stage presence. She commanded the stage in a way that I had not seen before. One of the things that stuck with me to this day is her confidence despite having significant cellulite. We were just starting to come out of the skinny ideal era, and I was just struck at how this stripper was boiling over with confidence.

The fella I was seeing became the pattern of all others. He was devoted to me, and I was losing interest. I do believe he might have been involved in dealing hard drugs. He had unexplained trips away and some odd messages on his answering machine that were coded. I was more suspicious when I found a baseball bat under his couch. Add to that, he wore dentures because all the teeth had been knocked out of his head.

We had been very close for the period I was in love with him, and he had a great sense of humour, but when I started distancing myself from him, he started getting weird/scary. I had decided to leave that city because I wanted to go to Florida and be a psychiatric nurse and a stripper. First, I wanted to return home and spend some time with my aging parents. I was on my way, but not before I had a dream about my boss and then approached him. That resulted in a trip away and sex. More looking for self-esteem.

10. Returning Home and Chaos

Ready for the trenches, yes? When I arrived back home, I stayed with my parents. The year was 2000. Before long, I bought a car and was soon working as a nurse at the hospital mental health unit. In those days I found myself attracted to a younger fella who was charismatic, athletic, and kept company with a popular group of friends. I will call him Charlie. He was quite charming at first. His mother was very rigid in her religious beliefs. I have anecdotally noticed, over the years, that instilling fear, guilt, and compliance into children's minds can come out sideways later on. I was raised in church, but it was not hell and brimstone theology.

We had some pretty good times, but everything changed once I had mentioned I was still planning on going to Florida. Charlie assaulted me, but I escaped from the car and ran with the keys barefoot down the road until I reached a hospital with a pay phone (I was barefoot because I was driving in bare feet). Charlie had been drinking, and I thought he was going to take the car and get into trouble. He had reached for the keys. I knew he had a very serious accident with a car before while drinking in a rage and no longer had a license. That night, two windows in my car were smashed. I tried to reason with Charlie for a brief period of time thinking things could get better. I learned that his brother was possibly more dangerous, having cut his girlfriend's brake lines in her car. He also assaulted someone in their eye orbit with a broken liquor glass, nearly costing them their sight.

One day, Charlie approached my parent's property, and my father, who was nearly ninety and typically quiet, yelled at him to get out of here. My mother said to me if my father had gotten his hands around his neck...

One afternoon, Charlie was confronting me on the sidewalk. It started with asking me if it was true that I heard voices. This was not clairvoyance, but it was a cleverly placed insult at the time. It targeted my *different* nature and possible comorbidity (loose use of the term) of mental illness in a shame-saturated question. I had never disclosed my history of anxiety or fear of psychosis to him. It would have been triggering for Charlie to unpack the reality that a person he considered inferior was leaving him. He needed to have control to salvage his pseudo self-esteem and save face with his friends. This was a **self-esteem crisis**—an irrefutable and tragic result of not answering the call to develop self-esteem successfully. It was challenging all the weak constructs in the place where self-esteem should be.

There are people who are in a friendly relationship with reality and acknowledge having low self-esteem and others who deny it, like Charlie. (I had been accosted by one of his friends who was saying Charlie had never acted like this before and "what had I done to him?" It was a witch hunt and females in that social group were supporting Charlie. I was blamed on the phone by one of them and rejected by all. (How dare an inferior person assert themselves against group norms especially when given a pass to be included in the first place). People walking were crossing the street because they knew it was an escalated situation. He pointed that out to me and threatened me in a few ways.

Another night, he held me hostage in my car all night. It became obvious this was not going to stop and I had to stay out of his reach. I was also trying to shelter my parents. I had to sleep in my car every night to get away from him. I changed locations every night covering great distances to find abandoned or secluded properties. My favourite place was an old abandoned house I had been inside before, but Charlie had a network of 'informants' with cars, so I didn't stay in one place twice. My car barely had a chance to cool off in those days. One night, I was driving and I saw Charlie walking. I knew he was looking for me. I recognized him from a distance and did a 180 degree turn in the road just in time. He started running after my car. Even though I was faster, it was terrifying to look in my rearview mirror and see him running after my car.

Everyday I was afraid to go anywhere where I might be trapped. He uttered threats to me more than once, and I went to a safe house for women. One morning, after a night shift at the hospital, I went out to my car and found the lock had been completely cored out of my door. I know it was him but of course had no proof. For the assault and threats, I involved police, and he was charged with assault and uttering threats. This was around the time of 9/11.

I continued to work while I was at the safe house. We had an admission for depression whom I will call Joe. Joe seemed very kind, and he was good looking. He flirted with me, and I was attracted to him. I thought I could help him, but I was selfishly looking to help myself.

After working a shift, I called the patient's phone and talked to him, inviting him out for a drive. He agreed, and we drove for hours longer than what he was allowed for his pass. Since Joe was late returning, there had been an alert made to the psychiatrist and his family. When he returned, he was scattered with his story about where he had been.

Joe was discharged from the hospital after a while, and I had my eyes opened by the house he said he owned. He lived in complete squalor. I didn't even know what a dust bunny was growing up in my parent's home. In this home, there were holes in the ceiling with a bird nest, dog feces in one of the closed off rooms, and a tarantula spider that had not been fed in who knows how long. I soon realized he also had a pot habit and was an alcoholic.

I set my mind on having some carpentry work done, helping the spider, cleaning, and helping Joe with his issues. I accomplished the physical issues with the house but had little success in helping him. I was, however, in love with him. I was also still thinking about conceiving, but now I decided I wanted to be a parent, and a good one.

One day when I was ovulating, I told Joe, and he said, "Let's go." Not long after, I woke up one morning with tender breasts, and I knew I was pregnant. I confirmed it with a pregnancy test. I was over the moon happy. My mother, however, did not share my excitement. Mom disliked this man/boy and said Joe would never look her straight in the eye. She was shaking when I told her. She eventually came on board with me giving him a chance. It surprised me when she shook his hand and said, "congratulations".

One night when I was a few months pregnant, I went out for a walk. I was observably pregnant. It was scary (I would use the word terrifying, but I think I have used my quota for that word in this book) to notice that Charlie was in a car that was following me. I sought safety in a store and called a cab to drive me home.

In the last trimester of the pregnancy, it became obvious Joe was not up for the challenge of getting himself straightened out. I left him even though I loved him. It was emotionally very hard, and I cried for days because I loved him and I had wanted it to work. I thought my baby had stopped moving inside me for over twenty-four hours and was terrified my emotional state had caused my baby to die. My mom reassured me that my baby was probably fine. I remember being in a grocery store within hours of my fright when I felt my baby move again. It was heaven. I had to look after myself to be a good parent to my baby, soon to be born. For the weeks before the delivery, there was no contact between Joe and myself.

11. My New Son and Life

When I was admitted for the birth of my son (2003), Mom was present, but I had denied Joe access to the event. After my son Calvin was born, I allowed Joe visitation at the hospital without me present in a visiting room. I was devastated about not being able to breastfeed. My breast reduction surgeon had assured me it would be possible, but the plumbing was just not there.

When I was discharged from the hospital, I stayed in my parent's home, although I had an apartment rented. I had a phone call from Joe, and I was in full agreement that he could visit, but I was not open to reconciliation. He said to me, "Don't fuck with me."

Within hours, I had a phone call from one of my colleagues at the hospital saying Joe had been admitted and had blown the whistle on me for taking him out on pass when he was a patient. Considering he was underemployed, I thought this was a desperate move on his part as I was the provider for the baby. The fall out was one I deserved. I abused my position of trust with someone who was vulnerable. I understand the gravity of what I did. I was fired from my job.

I was a devoted mom and never heard from Joe. Close to Calvin's first birthday, I saw an episode of Dr. Phil. He said that children who grow up without their fathers grow up with a hole in their heart in the shape of their father. Hearing that, I was moved emotionally, and I decided to invite Joe to Calvin's first birthday. He came and made regular visits. I still had feelings for him, but I kept them to myself.

I was able to secure a casual psychiatric nursing job in a hospital that would require me to move about two and a half hours from my childhood home. Joe started paying $100/month child support, which is absurdly low. I moved and began my job. Joe and I had another attempt at a relationship, but he continued to have the same kinds of issues.

There were two psychiatrists who worked at this hospital. One was Irish, and he enjoyed working with thought-disordered clients more than mood and personality disorders. He once said, behind the nursing station, that he "would like to put all the worried well in a dungeon". I find this comical and not offensive because, as you should know by now, I have a pass for the word 'crazy'.

12. Almost Murdered

During this time, Joe was nearly killed. I knew who the perpetrator was and that he had a very bad reputation and had been relocated under the witness protection act. I had also been told that Joe had shared naked pictures of the perpetrator's young adult daughter at a party.

Once, when I had been at Joe's, the perpetrator walked in the house, unannounced, and went straight to Joe's bedroom. I don't know what was said. I do know that it was threatening. I had been told he was a dangerous man and was involved in drugs.

Joe was hospitalized in ICU after the attempted murder, and it was uncertain whether he would live. He had deep gashes on his face, bruising over his whole body, a broken leg, and was in an induced coma being ventilated. It was savage. Joe had been lured to drink with the perpetrator at the perpetrator's house and then was assaulted and taken hostage in a vehicle to a destination where the perpetrator stood over him with a basketball-sized rock trained on his head. I learned the perpetrator's daughter was screaming at her father not to kill Joe.

Joe's brother maintains that the perpetrator had mistaken Joe for another person with the same name.

When my parents learned of the attempted murder, it was my father who seemed the most disgusted that I was still involved with Joe. My mom told me that if I knew what my father said about me I would never see him again.

After Joe was discharged from the hospital, he was in bad shape and needed considerable support. He lived with one of his brothers. There was a period where we still tried to make it work and tried to conceive more children, but it was not to be. Joe acted out in front of Calvin after I terminated the relationship, and he called me a robot. He recognized I had feelings for him and was leaving anyway. Allegedly, he smashed a picture of Calvin according to his brother who witnessed it. Calvin told me that Joe told him he would never see him again. Calvin reported Joe was telling him, "I [Laura] should be in jail". Joe's last words to me were, "I'll have the last laugh." My son has not seen Joe since then and that was the year 2007.

A bit of background about Joe as it was told to me by his brother. Joe had an extremely abusive father (Calvin's paternal grandfather). He apparently would cock a gun on Joe's mother's stomach when she was pregnant with Joe. Calvin's paternal grandfather was a high-achieving, good looking man but was very abusive. The paternal grandmother committed suicide by overdose when Joe was seventeen or eighteen. Mom told me that she was known to be a lovely woman. Joe identified strongly with being a victim in my opinion.

I was told the paternal grandfather died in 2017 in his home. He was not discovered for months.

13. Looking for a Good Man

Enter my drive to find a good father for Calvin and to have more children. I decided to join Match. I met two men who both seemed good. I was spending more time with one than the other because of geographical distance. Stephan was the fellow who I was most interested in and thought I had a future with. He lived quite close to me. On the nights when we were together, I continued my practice of co-sleeping with Calvin. I believed in the positive benefits of the "family bed." I had been an extremely devoted mom to Calvin and wanted to give him nurturing I never felt from my mom.

One night Calvin, almost four, sat up while I was giving Stephan a blow job. I saw his eyes were opened, but I had hoped nothing had registered. He laid back down and didn't say a word and seemed to immediately fall asleep.

I was sharing a good friendship with the other fella, James, who lived further away, and although I had told him "not to touch me" because I was not attracted to him, I still continued to see him. He seemed very interested in me. I was feeling positive and hopeful that something would work out for me but was mostly thinking in the direction of Stephan.

I felt it was reasonable to leave Calvin with Stephan while I went to work in those days. I was spending a lot of time with Stephan, and Calvin seemed happy in his company.

14. TERROR

A few days later, I was preparing for a shift. Calvin had a bath and went out to the couch. He said, "Mama, do you want to suck on my pee pee?" I thought that was alarming, and I asked him to come talk to me. In sheer panic, on my knees in front of him, I asked him if Stephan had ever sucked on his pee pee, and he excitedly said "Yes, yes" and pointed to a little calendar I had on the wall for him and said, "This day, this day!!!"

With all my mental problems to that date, I had never felt my blood run cold before, but it did in that instant, and I will never forget it. He must have perceived my terror, and with me saying, "No one is ever supposed to do that to you," he ran and hid in the closet. He had never done that before in his life.

I was out of my mind and called in sick and called my best friend, Angelina, and Stephan. Stephan came to my apartment and said we could call the police if I wanted. I said we would hold off on that, but we had to talk to a counselor. We arranged for that, and protocol required a report to child protection services.

Child protection could not find enough evidence, so it was dismissed. I insisted that Stephan have a polygraph test, and he agreed to that. I met with the polygraph examiner and learned how the test would proceed. While it was being conducted, I waited in my car with Calvin. Still very agitated about everything, I was quizzing Calvin about times he was with Stephan. He said, "Such a small pee pee for such a big man." That supply of detail undermined my confidence in an innocent polygraph test result and went straight to my stomach. Once the test was over, I was told that Stephan passed.

I had my family saying that it was my fault for allowing the co-sleeping, and others were saying that I had asked Calvin leading questions. Stephan's family seemed like good people, so I had periods of confusion. My best friend, Angelina, also said she did not think anything had happened. The relationship was not able to survive that even though he was never charged.

I gradually put the issue behind me and started leaning on James. I was very cautious to say the least, but he was patient and started to win me over. He was on board with the idea of having children. At this time, I also found out that my fallopian tubes had become blocked with progressive endometriosis. We started researching IVF therapy and learned James' work insurance would mostly cover the treatment costs. We were married in my parent's house, and it was the last time my dad was in the house before he passed. He was in a nursing home at that point and had a day pass for the wedding. He was such a good man and set a good example for me. I know my parents were relieved to have me married, and I imagine they could only hope the marriage would last. It was the summer of 2007.

A few short months after the marriage began, my dad was in the advanced stages of dilated cardiomyopathy. My mom called me and said I should come home. I loved my dad dearly despite anything he could have thought of me. He asked me to prepare what was his last meal. He requested that I go home and make him some scrambled eggs. I was so happy to be able to do something for him.

After I returned with the eggs and he ate, he said, "We had our problems." I told him how much I was going to miss him, and he said he was going to miss me too. He stopped eating and his care became palliative. He did not suffer long. I attended his funeral, but my mom would not let me attend the internment in the spring. My mom wore a black leather skirt to the funeral, which caught the attention of Shelly but not me. Hearing the hymn *In the Garden* played on the pipe organ with choir accompaniment in the large sanctuary was overwhelming. I made a shrine for him. When I think of him, it is with pride and love.

When I think of James, it is true he could be funny by spells, but we were never really close the way I wanted to be. Curiously, when I would try to get his input on serious things, I always found his responses were unrelated for lack of a better way to describe it. His answers were off-the-wall and detached from what I was communicating about with him.

He was consistent about this. Sometimes I felt like he was speaking to me in riddles. He also had a peculiar habit of *quasi pretending* he heard words differently. I say this because I am sure he was not hearing impaired. For example, if I said I was going to the store he would repeat back, "You're going outdoors". Once, when I had wanted to be close, I suggested he pick a slow song, and he selected some kind of formal waltz. Perhaps his mind was elsewhere or he could not be close in that way. I stopped asking his input unless I felt I really needed to.

One area where I thought he had wisdom was in his attitude that people will stay true to themselves. He captured this perfectly when he used to say, "Mom is doing Mom things" or "Calvin is doing Calvin things." This made me think that he was not imposing expectations on the nature of others. However, there are some additional things I am keeping to myself that now make me believe he gaslit our entire relationship.

At one point during the marriage, I was attracted to another woman. This woman was also very masculine, and I was the first to let her know I found her attractive. We went for a drive one day, and because I was feeling very attracted to her, my driver's side window steamed up. I asked James if I could explore more with her, and he was completely against it, so I distanced myself from her.

James and I conceived twins through IVF. I was very excited to be pregnant with a boy and girl. They were born in 2008. My son, Mingus, had a birth defect. I had a hard time dealing with it at first. Amber was so sweet and wanted to bond from the beginning. When we came home from the hospital, I felt that Calvin was being ignored by James, and I had significant trouble with that. It was a fear of mine that James would push Calvin to the side.

At the same time, my mother went to the hospital for a hemiglossectomy because of tongue cancer. She had never smoked and was not a drinker. I felt she had developed cancer because of stress. Her life since childhood had been filled with stress, and I had been an enormous worry for her. At the hospital, my mom commented, "These are real nurses."

TERROR

I had read a book, many years before, that documented the power of mind over matter. There was a man who had been diagnosed with terminal cancer and had developed a meditation to help himself. He imagined his immune system had wolves that would scan his body for rats (cancer) and would sniff them out and break their necks. I told her about this and tried to encourage her to meditate before she ever got to the point of needing the radical surgery. The cancer continued. She was considered a good candidate for surgery. Although it was a serious surgery, I was expecting a good outcome.

Initially, post op, she seemed to be recovering, but then she had some unexpected post-surgery complications. When Calvin visited her, she held his hand. He was like an angel to her. She also smiled on Mingus and Amber. In an attempt to influence the marriage, she asked James to shave before he kissed me, and she asked me to close the cupboard doors for him. Mom didn't want me looking crazy. Mom said she did not want to go to a nursing home, and I reassured her she could live with us. I was willing to move mountains to accommodate her. She gave me the family cottage that day. She was communicating on a notepad. Still feeling confident, I went home briefly to take a breather and look after the twins, who were about two months old. Within a few short hours, a cascade of more serious complications resulted in her having a heart attack and her kidneys shutting down while she was on full life support.

When the doctor told me that her kidneys were not perfusing and I knew she was still getting IV fluids and there was nothing more they could do, I wanted them to urgently stop her suffering. I can't put into words how desperately I wanted them to stop her support in that very instant so she would not suffer another second.

I could not have loved my mom any more than I did. I absolutely believe she did the best she could. She dedicated herself to protecting me and trying to nurture me to the best of her ability. Her intentions spoke to me louder than any mistakes she could have made. I have nothing but eternal love, respect and a feeling of sadness for her. I objectively know she may have contributed to my problems but people are humans with limitations. I will defend her until I die. They could not have chained me to the room when she was "quickly going downhill" after they withdrew support. I would like to believe I could have the strength to stay with her now so she was not alone, but I couldn't handle her dying then. I was utterly dependent on her even though we had conflict over everything. Mom (2008) and Dad (2007) passed within eleven months of one another. I am extraordinarily protective of the special things she left me. I feel close to her through them.

15. The Bottom of the Mental Illness Barrel

During the initial days of grieving, in November 2008, James' mother and sister came over to visit. I could hear them laughing and carrying on in the kitchen. I felt intense rage. I refused to come upstairs.

James and I started having difficulties around this time, and we separated for a bit, and he took the twins to his sister's over Christmas. Calvin stayed with me. The following is no midlife crisis. Sometimes I wonder if it all happened because I didn't forward some chain Facebook post on to ten other people. Smile.

Unaware I was becoming psychotic, I started noticing that many things were extremely funny that would not normally be funny. This was late December 2008. "Psychosis is a loss of contact with reality where a person may experience delusions (false beliefs) or hallucinations (seeing, hearing, or smelling things that others do not)" (National Institute of Mental Health). Things that didn't even make sense were new and exciting and had special meaning. I was not realizing I was tipping into psychosis but was mostly feeling I had better perception and importance.

I reached out to my eccentric laughing buddy from junior high and described elaborate drawing ideas for him to try. They were from delusions I had about cars with flames and other detailing. It did not take him long to block me. If there was one person who I believed would have 'forgiven' my psychosis, it was him, but after accepting my friend request post psychosis, I feel I was only tolerated.

Delusions are hard for people to understand. I can't explain it any better than a person believes these things to be true the same way you believe the ground is under your feet. I did not hear voices, but I did have some hallucinations. I remember many of my delusions and things I did.

I believed the colour indigo was illegal. Calvin had a rubber ball that was the illegal colour and I stabbed it to get rid of it. It is interesting that indigo and pink are my actual favourite colours. I started posting dating profiles seeking millionaires and then talked in grandiose form about what we would do together. I had one person respond, and I called the cops to come see evidence that he was stalking me. When the cop arrived, he reviewed the correspondence and said he felt the man was just interested.

I started believing that the local radio personalities had "sharpened their teeth" in the photographs online for the radio's webpage. I went to the dentist around this time and he was telling me about a local news story where someone had been stabbed. I felt he was telling me because it had special relevance to me. I thanked him for telling me. I also believed he left a sharp edge on my tooth so that I would continue to think about him.

As the psychotic days rolled on, I had a very distinct delusion that I was a human mirror. I had a notion that people could interact with me and see themselves.

James saw my dating profile and said he was feeling jealous and returned home in January 2009. I thought he looked like a muppet when he returned and spent a lot of time laughing about that. I don't know what was going on in his head about me, but I was now going out driving and thought I had a mission to find abusive men. I was interested in purchasing a gun. I identified two such men and chastised one man for driving an orange car as I believed that was a dead giveaway he was abusive. I saw another man in a parking lot and made threatening gestures toward him.

Despite being psychotic, I was still able to function to some degree. I ordered Chinese takeout one evening, and I reported for my nursing shift that night. Once I was on duty in the nursing unit, I thought Calvin's father had planted a patient on the unit to watch me. I laughed hysterically over some tomato juice that represented blood to me. The unit manager came in that evening, which was unusual. She talked to me for a bit but then left.

The Bottom of the Mental Illness Barrel

I assume one of my colleagues had called the unit manager in, noticing I was acting strange. That was my last shift because I was required to see occupational health before returning, and I obviously did not pass the screen. I remember the appointment, and I was believing strange things about the decor in the occupational health nurses' office. I was far more interested in the messaging I was picking up on from her decor as opposed to anything that was being talked about.

One day James and I went out for a drive. My Tercel had an aftermarket stereo and 12-inch sub, so favourite songs like *Gimme All Your Lovin'* by ZZ Top, *Disturbia by* Rhianna, *and Right Round by* Flo Rida, to name a few, were expanding my mood further. We went to Starbucks, and I still believed I was on my mission to find abusive men. I was very disinhibited. Feeling I had identified one, I walked up to him and kissed him aggressively when he was standing in line. He said to me afterward, "Next time we do it on my time." Even though I was psychotic, I recognized he was responding to my aggression and was promising the same in return.

I had found another man who I thought was a problem and closed his laptop. He opened it and I closed it again. He then said to James, "You need to put that thing on a leash." I had never seen James blush before, but he did then and said we needed to leave.

I had a meltdown over Goldfish crackers and coffee cream. I asked James to pick up flavoured fish crackers and plain coffee cream and he came back with plain fish crackers and flavoured coffee cream. I cried and cried about it and was also angry. I was crying uncontrollably in the shower, and he actually came into the shower to comfort me, clothes and all.

I started wearing sunglasses in the house to stop me from "burning bushes" in the yard with my eyes. I believed there were monkeys in the woods that were waving sticks at me because I was not good enough to be human and was not good enough to be a monkey. I believed there were First Nations people outside the house blowing smoke in through the windows from a peace pipe, and I had the hallucination of being able to smell it. One funny delusion I had was the belief the government had put rubber in the pavement and scattered rubber over roads to make cars more bouncy. But wait... I might still think this is a fun idea.

I thought the history channel was showing me information that I needed to know to take my place in the world. I believed I could blind James by looking into his eyes. I believed James could telepathically communicate with the babies. I had a hallucination that I had burned snake eyes into his neck and could see the two dots. I also believed I was causing another ice age and the snow plows were being made larger and larger in response. I believed Jennifer Hudson had written the song "Spotlight" for me. I also believed I had been personally invited to appear on the Ellen DeGeneres Show. The home I had grown up in was somewhat of a *brick house*. I believed the brick face was a screen for my mom, where she hid a secret affinity toward black people. I believed she was representative of the type of woman identified in the song. I also had days that I called 'opposite' days, which bent my mind further. In one hospital, I wrote that it was opposite day on the patient white board. Opposite Day on the psych unit! I can't even imagine how psychotics together, on a locked unit, spool each other up.

One day, I was in the city core trying to offer street people advice and money. I wanted to recruit an 'army' of muscle to confront pedophiles. I had elevated any compromised person to a superior status. I was nearly hit by a bus that day, and a street person came out of his stupor to protect me. He waved his arms at me and said, "Be careful! You were almost hit by that bus!"

One morning when James was at work, I carried Calvin out to the school bus in my arms and "delivered" him to the school bus driver. (I had already arranged for the bus stop to be changed to our property, citing I was being stalked). I believed this would protect him from pedophiles. I started thinking that I needed to baptize the twins to protect them from pedophiles. It was winter, and I turned the heat up in the house to bust and opened the front and back doors.

I called a minister and told her what I was doing, and she arrived at the house after I had finished bathing the twins. Amber had front teeth that had erupted, and before the minister arrived, I carefully rubbed my finger back and forth on a tooth until it bled. I believed this would protect her from pedophiles. When the minister arrived, she called James to come home from work. She took me to the hospital, one where I didn't work.

For the entire drive, I sat with my head between my knees. I thought my head was on a spigot and that we were going to crash land and I was supposed to impale myself for my mistakes. It was terrifying. Once I got to the hospital, I was admitted. I was very paranoid and singing "Jesus Loves Me". When they walked me up to the unit, I saw dinner plates on the floor and had a strong compulsion to throw them like frisbees. I was in a high observation room for a spell. I believed James controlled the airspace above the hospital and it was going to be evacuated with only me left inside and then bombed.

I met a female patient whom I felt a connection to. I felt I had met my soul sister and gave her my mom's diamond engagement ring. I wanted to be close to her as a friend, and the ring was a symbol of that. I was later told she was a prostitute.

One day I thought I had to die to save my children. I put a plastic bag over my head and thought to myself that if I was found, it meant I was supposed to live, and if not, I was supposed to die.

I do remember nurses coming in, and then I was transported by ambulance to a different hospital. The ambulance ride was terrifying to me as I believed if I did not think pure thoughts I was going to go out the back of the ambulance on the stretcher onto the highway.

In that hospital, I had someone sitting outside my room the entire time. This was the hospital where I had gone for an intake assessment for my eating disorder while in university. I was very preoccupied with some OCD-type undoing rituals that I made up as I went along—sequenced steps and unwinding steps, organizing and balancing things. There was a black female on the unit, and I told her to stay away from me because I was racist. She said to me that she didn't believe I was. I had a delusion that the sound of bells ringing were people experiencing orgasm. At some point, I was brought back to the original hospital. I realized my mistake in giving my mom's engagement ring away and luckily the nurses had noticed and recovered it for me. I must have been doing somewhat better as I was no longer an involuntary patient and they discussed my discharge. I said I was not going to take medication, and when I left, I was driven home by taxi. James said he did not want me there and had taken the children, so I packed the car with all my favourite glass ornaments from my mom, family picture albums and paper, and left for the family cottage three hours away. I was observing the weather as I drove and believing I had caused it. Once I arrived at the cottage community, I saw someone I knew changing his car headlights and I thought this was directly in response to the weather I was causing.

At the cottage, I started thinking that my parents had bought me a seaside insane asylum anticipating I was going to go crazy. It was odd that I seemed to have that little bit of insight. The other hint of insight I had was I believed I had "psychosis" glasses. I was posting about my psychosis glasses on Facebook. It proves what Nathaniel Branden said about the mind "somewhere there is knowledge." I am not suggesting any people who are psychotic will have any degree of insight.

I believed I was a personal relationship counselor to Britney Spears. I believed that people in magazines could see me back. I believed cars were alive and could see me, especially when they were in reverse. I thought my car acknowledged me. When I was at the cottage, I planned to assault James with a fire poker if he showed up.

One psychotic day, I was thinking about the most eccentric person I knew. I could see clearly he was the King of the Storybook people, so I made a short pilgrimage to his vacant property and spent time on his lawn. *Remembering him in my lucid mind as I write this*, I will offer my impression of him. He was a professor (of course) and had the complete list of eccentric identifiers. He piled cardboard to the ceiling, his window dressings were in shreds, he wore ill-fitting, tattered clothing, played an organ in the middle of the night, and he had to be reminded it was time to go when visiting others. He had a convertible, and the top didn't work. Once, he drove a long distance in a rainstorm with a shower curtain tied around his head. He hosted the most unusual parties where he would put a roast in the oven when the party began and made up his own games for party guests. He was unable to maintain electricity at the property in later years.

His property had once been the crowning glory of the community, situated close to the ocean. His parents hosted proper garden parties. One day, long before I had psychosis, my friend Tim, the professor, and I went to the playground a short walk away. We discovered the hardware on the swingset needed lubricant and somehow, together, accomplished the task of finding a ladder and applying heavy grease. We spent most of the time laughing. I believe this level of eccentricity, as seen in the professor, imparts minimal insight but, I felt, in that playful afternoon, he might have joined us in laughing at ourselves. Which I think was remarkable—madness observing itself. Perhaps this was facilitated by feeling safe and not judged negatively. If there is a slot between psychosis and reality this degree of eccentricity pushes the limit. If I could name it, it is a low level madness, kind of like hydroplaning on reality. I think the DSM-5 calls it, unceremoniously, Cluster A.

I was talking about this book with Tim the other day and he reminded me of a psychosis story I had forgotten. Somewhere along the line, I had picked up a social worker. He said one day I had met him at his cottage and I was trying to convince him to call her and tell her I was ok. He didn't feel it was the best thing to do, but he gave me his word, some Oreos, and sent me on my way.

At the cottage, I felt a compulsion to rate people according to how well or sick they were mentally. One day, while delusional, I went to a local farm that sold fresh eggs and milk. I had always thought the lady who sold the eggs 'acted crazy', so I thought I needed to go there. I bought some eggs, left a sarcastic five-dollar tip, and returned to the cottage where I promptly smashed all the eggs at once on the back concrete step.

Another day, I went to a local business where developmentally challenged individuals were employed. It was a laundromat and bakery business. One of the employees invited me to a social event, and it almost brought me to tears to be invited, and, more importantly, accepted.

I decided to go to the hospital to prove I was not ill to a psychiatrist. When I presented at the hospital, I was heckling a nurse while waiting to be seen. Heckling her for being normal, if you will. I also was insisting I wanted to only see a psychiatrist and not the triage doctor.

I decided to leave before I was assessed. I stopped at a gas station for gas and they alerted the police about me because I could not sign my Visa slip because of some surveillance idea. The police found me a few hundred feet before the cottage and parked behind my Tercel. They were trying to get me out of my car, and I was refusing until I had talked to a lawyer. Negotiations continued, and they mentioned a spiked track, but once I heard them talking about breaking a window I said I would get out if they allowed me to talk to my lawyer first. They did not keep their end of the deal and handcuffed me straight away. My best friend Angelina and her mom were watching helplessly from her mom's cottage porch as I was stuffed into the cruiser. It was the off-season, so nobody else saw the circus.

When they transported me to the hospital, I felt more agitated about saving my children. I was screaming and spitting at everyone, since I perceived they were trying to stop me. I was still in handcuffs, and the police were bending my thumbs backward to try and subdue me. It was extremely painful. Staff were wearing face shields around me, and all I could think of was saving my children. They clearly gave me an injection because I woke up on the psych unit the next day, in the care of my old colleagues. I am guessing the injection medication was Accuphase. I think the drug manufacturers were having fun when they named this big gun. Accuphase sounds a bit like an outer space themed chemical restraint.

I was hospitalized for a time again and was not swallowing (cheeking) my medication. I remember fighting with cleaning staff because I had taken one of their trolleys and was using it as an office to keep my notes safe. I told the psychiatrist I was a better parent 'on paper', with 'my marbles scattered all over the place', than James. I had bolted from the unit and was trying to escape, only to be captured by security. Over time, perhaps the structure of the hospital stabilized me and returned a bit of my lucidity, or at least enough of it that I was able to be made a voluntary patient. I requested a discharge, insisting I needed to mow the lawn at the cottage. I was trying to be responsible toward the property. I had already been told by my real estate agent that the lawn at my mom's house was like a hayfield. The discharge was granted against medical advice.

I once again returned to the insane asylum by the water and quickly decompensated. I believed my parents were at war inside me. This was in May 2009. This time I left there and asked my friend Angelina if I could stay with her at her home. She was agreeable. I had the idea that I could get ahead of time and the way to do it was to send continuous faxes. I was sending them to the pharmacy. (Time travel through a fax machine—sounds right). Angelina was such a gentle person and so good. She didn't confront me but gently persuaded me that the fax was for her husband's work. I only have a scanner in our home. (grin)

The Bottom of the Mental Illness Barrel

One rather funny thing that occurred with the psychosis happened in a random lawyer's office. I presented at reception and made a plea that I had an urgent matter that I needed to talk to a lawyer about. The receptionist made special arrangements for me to see the lawyer. I went in with a notebook that I had been writing in and the required personal identification. Sitting across from the lawyer, I asked if I could borrow his scissors. He gave them to me, and I cut a page in half with a zigzag pattern. I then asked him to legally make a statement, committed to paper, that the piece cut away belonged to the original page, and to notarize it. He told me to "get out". I think he thought I was trying to make a mockery of him, but I felt it was vitally important. I left. When I think back to it I still laugh.

At another point, I started feeling like I was homicidal and felt very impulsive about it. I had no plan, just the feeling. I couldn't figure out for what reason, but it was intense and terrifying, so I drove myself up to the emergency department and was lying on the floor begging for help to stop me. The ER nurse reminded me that I was a nurse at that hospital and told me to stop. The response was odd in that the psychiatrist who assessed me prescribed medication, released me, and made a comment about how terrible a thing schizophrenia was.

As quickly and mysteriously as it appeared, the homicidal impulse left on its own, but I started calling 911 and human rights reporting pedophiles abusing my children. It was around the time when the elementary school had the yearly family picnic, and I was calling the school and asking how they could let pedophiles attend a school family picnic.

I found my way into a safe house for women. The facility was a historic property. I remember thinking the clothing hooks in the hall were meat hooks. I had an olfactory hallucination in that house, and it came and went. It was very strange and unforgettable. I believed I was not good enough to unload the dishwasher that had children's dishes inside. I was kicked out, with them saying I was 'sick'.

One day, I was driving and picked up a man who was walking. I asked him if he wanted a drive. He was going to the bank. I wanted to go to the bank machine, too, but I was very paranoid about surveillance. I asked him if he wanted to go to the casino. He must have perceived something wrong with me and he declined. That was probably very lucky for me. He did accept a drive to his home from me. When we got there, he asked if I wanted to come inside. I was thinking about it, but when I looked at his front door, I saw a huge smearing of blood (hallucination) so I passed.

Again, I went to a hospital, and when I was in the ER, I was trying to reach the Irish psychiatrist at the hospital where I had worked. I got his voicemail. I was asking for his help to get me out and telling him that he was eccentric, too. He had a habit of stuffing unwrapped food, including cookies or anything else he could scrounge, into his sports jacket pockets like a street person, or eating leftovers from patient trays. Sometimes he had body odor which was not attractive. Rumor said his house was a chaotic mess. He was wickedly funny and good looking, and I was definitely crushing on him (he just needed a bath, new clothes, and a house clean). He did have an air of superiority, and had a tendency to dominate conversations by speaking over others. I tried to tone down the way he engaged my humor, not wanting to appear so transparent, and also feeling some degree of shame because others laughed at him when he left the nursing station. Maybe I was more interesting to him as a psychotic.

I was assessed and transported by the cops to another hospital. The cops stopped by a drive-thru coffee place and offered to buy me a drink. I asked for tea. I was not handcuffed, and there was an opening between the back seat where I was and where the two cops in front were. It took everything in me not to throw the hot tea at them. One of the first things I thought after I became lucid again was that cops should never take chances with people who are psychotic. I wish police forces knew this, and I think this exact thing every time I pass that police station. Behavior from acute psychosis cannot be predicted, in my opinion.

When I was admitted to the new hospital, I had a lot of paranoia and laid on the floor for some type of grounding. I was also licking the windows. I was terrified. I had a roommate who I addressed as soon as I arrived in the room. I promptly told her I was sicker than any cat lady. I think she purposefully pissed on the floor. I asked the nurses to remedy the cat urine smell, and they told me I should have that discussion with her myself. We later became buddies. We both stashed items that might be of some future use and organized them on our nightside tables. On one occasion, there was a male patient who looked at my mom's engagement ring and said it was nice. I sucker punched him in the face for it. They called a code white and convinced me to take more medication or I would have to go to the locked high observation room. I was also prevented from calling 911 anymore. I called my lawyer a few times.

I was in that hospital for a long time. I remember my attending psychiatrist discussing with me changing medication from Seroquel to a higher potency antipsychotic, Olanzapine. I think this was following the night I was saying some very disinhibited sexual things to the security guard. I also remember that she was irritated by me using her first name.

I started to get better. For timeline purposes, this was when Micheal Jackson died in the summer of 2009. Then came the good news of supervised visits with my children in the hospital. As my psychosis was lifting, my bulimia started. I was ecstatic to see Calvin when he came. I had started saving up little things that I knew would be of interest to him. When Amber and Mingus came, I was so overjoyed to see them but so deeply saddened that they did not know me.

16. Lucid and Not Good

When I was discharged, James reluctantly took me back. I found out later from Joe's family that James tried to give Calvin back to Joe. It broke my heart, but I know Joe was not capable/willing to take on the responsibility of his son. I already felt from videos I saw when I was hospitalized that James was not interested in Calvin. I needed the family together and needed to be a parent.

Looking back and thinking about how schizophrenia tends to present in late adolescence, it is no surprise my psychotic flight from reality happened when I had lost my lifeline, my mom. As I mentioned, we had lots of conflict, but I was very dependent on her. Her death was the end of my symbolic adolescence and launchpad into adulthood without the necessary skill set.

17. INFERIOR TO THE 9TH DEGREE

Enter the depression of my life. I can't begin to tell you how depressed I was when I was discharged. I felt subhuman. I can't think of any other way to put it. It was almost like the delusion I had when I was psychotic where I was not good enough to be a human and not good enough to be an animal. I felt so beneath every other human and could not accept how defective I was. I could not convey the shame and feelings of inferiority I felt.

I had a lot of suicidal ideation but no plan. I cried and cried every day, and I was terrified of the psychosis returning. It was torture. I was constantly checking my reality orientation in more than three spheres. Normal testing would be person, place, and time. During those days, James told me that his work had a retinal security scan. I could not figure out whether believing that would make me delusional or was proof that I was delusional. It was beyond distressing to me, and I asked my psychiatrist about it. To this day, I don't know whether it was true or if James was playing with my head. I was scared to go for any walks or drives beyond the grocery store. I missed my mom very badly but was glad she was not witnessing everything that had happened. I could barely speak to people. I tried to return to my job, but I was dissociating at work and had to stop. Parenting was a struggle because I was so paralyzed by depression and feelings of inferiority. I was on the couch all the time and parented from there. I would try to get my toddler twins to come to me so that I could at least hold them on the couch and they could experience physical closeness to me. I tried to get James to cover for me by insulting him and telling him he paid more attention to the dog than the children. My thought process was that I couldn't do it, but maybe I could shame him into shouldering more responsibility. He said, "I never thought I would hear you say that".

People with mental illness seem to universally want to be off medication to prove to themselves that they are somehow ok. I was no different. Mental illness is already so damaging to self-esteem that pills represent one more layer of not being good enough. In the hospital, I was taking Olanzapine 15 mg at bedtime. Soon after I was discharged, I titrated down my medication until I was at 2.5 mg. I did this despite my fear of a second break. I already knew that after a first break the threshold for a subsequent break was lower. I wanted to feel some relief from feeling subhuman.

I was not allowed to take an antidepressant because it could tip me back into mania and then psychosis... happiness by medication was contraindicated, surely a weakness in the medical model. Interestingly, my new regular psychiatrist had been a colleague in the hospital where I had worked as a RN. One of his first statements to me was that I had been "floridly" psychotic. I was diagnosed as having bipolar type 1 with psychosis. I had just about everything in the DSM-5 (Diagnostic and Statistical Manual of Mental Disorders). Feel free to add personality disorder to the pile. I was not diagnosed as such, but I realize I have some cluster B traits, and, to be *safe*, A features. At any rate, the overlap is redundant at some point.

I reached out to my deceased mom's friend who was in her 90's. She was so kind and encouraging to me. She fielded daily crying phone calls from me. Once, she said it was a shame my twins had been born, but she was motivated to help me. I primarily wanted her to somehow jumpstart my parenting abilities. I also reached out to my cousins because I had no siblings. They felt I was too much and turned their backs on me. I was needy for sure. I wanted to get support so I could parent better and feel something other than feeling like a defective animal. I struggled with them not helping me when I really needed support. My mom had helped them in personal ways. My cousin Shelly lost her mom when she was only seventeen and my mom had been a special aunt to her. Add to that she was a RN and she had been remembered in my mom's will. I was very alone in my unique struggle to put myself back together.

I limped along with my terrible self-esteem and dread of becoming ill again for many years inside the family and failed my children. I gained a terrific amount of weight trying to soothe myself. I felt so desperately low that I could not even fantasize because I was not even worthy of that given how inferior and defective I was. In the past, I had enjoyed a rich romantic fantasy life, but I could not fantasize at all. You have to be at least human status to attract the attention of another human being even in fantasy. I had a recurring dream for years that I had almost finished fourth year university and could not finish my nursing program. I had this exact same dream almost nightly. My poor self-esteem even followed me in my dreams.

18. DISCOVERY

Around 2015, I had started to get counseling to help me be a better mom. I felt that I needed to be better for my children, especially Amber and Mingus. I had also thought I should foster a relationship between Calvin and his father. James had never been close to Calvin, and it seemed time that Calvin at least be in contact with Joe. I was starting to feel stronger.

I also felt Joe should be paying more child support, and that was increased by court order to $230/month. He had said to me before that he was only going to work part time because he did not want to pay more child support. (When Calvin was still a toddler, he said he would go to jail before paying anything retroactive, the same day I was looking for a job).

I wanted supervised visits, if they were to happen, based on his acting out when I had left him for the last time. This angered him, and he said he reported me to the hospital that I had most recently worked at for my conduct over how we first met. It surprised me that he would do that so many years later, not understanding that hurting me financially was not in the best interest of his son. At any rate, I had already closed the door on my nursing career.

Joe did not see Calvin but maintained some text contact after that time. I believe he loved Calvin, but he perceived slights where there were none. Any hint of rejection and he couldn't handle it and retreated into being a victim and vindictiveness. My mother always said he and his siblings were "fight cats."

Discovery

I can remember asking James if he could give Calvin a bit more attention and his response was that it should happen naturally. One evening, I asked James to tell Calvin it was suppertime. Calvin was in the bathroom and old enough that he needed privacy. James got mad that Calvin was not listening and unlocked the door. I heard Calvin scream at him to get out. I was quite unhappy about this and confronted James. He complained that Calvin did not listen to him and that people at work did not listen to him.

James *could* be funny, and he had some good traits, for sure. One funny thing he said about Mingus' energy was, "Mingus should have a hamster wheel". When deciding to get Calvin a dirt bike, because of his cautious nature, I asked about Mingus wanting one when he was older. James said we could get Mingus one without an engine. He also called Mingus "Calvin's agent/lawyer", since Mingus was always promoting anything Calvin wanted. I wouldn't even have my eyes open yet in the morning, and Mingus would be hammering something at me to benefit Calvin. One day Mingus came upstairs with a piece of paper taped to his shirt, with the correct spelling and correct messaging that read "boss/manager". We laughed when Mingus came home from a friend's house with three rocks and an "asteroid". I can't resist the next one. There was a time when Mingus was *against* gravy. One week he announced, "Gravy is yucky for me". That was followed by, "I am allergic to gravy". Apparently, I was not getting the message because the final thing he said was, "Gravy is poisonous for me". One day, we were at Toys"R"Us and Amber saw an enderman stuffie from Minecraft. She said, "Oh Mom, that is the enderman that's been chasing Dad!" Jenna also told me, "Mom, when I was in your belly, I saw three ocelots (Minecraft cats)". Children say the cutest things possible. James was absolutely there for homework support and sports activities, and was even a coach for hockey. He was agreeable to most of the home improvement ideas I suggested, and we had a heated pool that we enjoyed with the children. We also had memorable experiences at the cottage. I can't ever remember arguing with him much. The sweet cat was never a fan of James.

In those days, I started wondering about James and what he had been up to. I suppose some of that was guilt because in reality, I offered James very little. I can own this. James would have had to be stupid to not perceive my lack of interest in him, and most men want sex, affection, and praise. Homer McDonald, who I reference later, says that praise is often more important than sex. I didn't have to look farther than Facebook to see that he was having some degree of a relationship online. It really shook me up. Although I wasn't in love with him, I had tried to remain loyal to him, even when approached by the sexiest male from the private school I attended so many years ago. When I declined the schoolmate's offer, he said, "As you wish". Those are very powerful words. They convey self-assurance, respect for boundaries, and zero neediness to have one's own way. Convincing would have come from a weak position. There were no flies on him, and this relaxed response was consistent with his personality. I certainly wanted to meet him, but my integrity was more important.

In light of the new Facebook evidence, my immediate decision was if James was unfaithful, I was going to be, too, and I was going to be open about it. I was not in love with him, so I could not think of a reason why I should be faithful if he wasn't. I confronted him. He emphatically told me he didn't want to lose me and started falling all over me. It was nice that he wanted to keep me, but I had made my mind up. I thought I better get with the current times and upgraded from a flip phone to a smartphone so I could have a dating profile on my phone. I also started dieting, which quickly led to the reemergence of my eating disorder.

Having grown older, I was at increased risk for secondary problems because of purging. Bread was one of my favourite things to binge on, and because it was completely undigested when I purged, there was terrific force and volume. I can remember when I created a hernia in my esophagus. The pain was incredible. I knew from reading, if it ruptured, it could be life-threatening. Everytime I went to the bathroom to purge, I wondered if I would be alive afterward, so on a daily basis I felt like I could die.

I had a scope done and learned that food was freely passing between my stomach and esophagus in the wrong direction because of an insufficient cardiac sphincter, which would normally keep food in the stomach. It was severe reflux. My sphincter was damaged from forceful vomiting.

The consequence of this was a couple times I aspirated food while sleeping and developed chemical pneumonia. As you can imagine, stomach acids and food do not belong in the lungs. I have scar tissue from that, diagnosed by a CAT scan.

With my openness about dating and being on my smartphone all the time, James became extremely attentive toward me. There were days when I received two bouquets of flowers in one day. It was to such a degree that I felt he was invested in our relationship. I said I was willing to change direction and be monogamous even though I was not in love with him.

Around this time, I had developed a stuttering problem. What was more curious was that James and Calvin started stuttering as well. It seemed to have a contagion about it that was exacerbated by shame we all seemed to experience over it. It was not as intense as the feeling I had in my late twenties where I felt if I spoke at all my words would be garbled, but it was bad.

It was not longer than two weeks after I committed to being monogamous that the attentiveness from James started dropping off. I thought once again, I could not trust him. I did not announce my departure from the monogamy agreement and reactivated my dating profile.

19. Out of My League

I met a man who I believed was well out of my league. I will call him Tyler. I can honestly say he is the type of man that women throw themselves at. Initially, he had set out to have fun. I felt Tyler was a safe bet because we were both sexually clean and he had regular HIV testing done for his work. He was incredibly sexy, self-assured, and happy, although he was married. He was also an excellent father to his children and inspired me to go farther with my children. He had a great sense of humour. He was an excellent stick driver and I allowed him to drive the (disappointingly automatic) Lexus IS 350 I had at the time. I thought it was a nice-looking car. (It was atomic silver, which was a great color for the design). James was not allowed to drive it. I really couldn't afford the car. Even though I take care of things, my test for affording something is not being paranoid about taking care of those things. It was heartbreaking to wake up and find it vandalized and intuitively knowing it was the work of Charlie. The Tercel has permanent Charlie branding, as well. Tyler knew I favored the Tercel, and the Tercel had less things that could go wrong. Tyler took Calvin and I off-roading in the Jeep, at my request, because I was excited we were going to go up a vertical hill I thought exceeded the limits of the vehicle.

Tyler has some degree of erectile dysfunction, but I was so enamoured by him that I was able to put that aside. The more I fell in love with him, however, the more it bothered me. I knew he was also in love with me. I perceived it as a problem of me not being enough of a turn on for him.

When I felt him backing off, it hit me hard. I did the only thing I knew what to do, which was to introduce some competition. I activated my online dating profile again. I was hurting. I was hurting so bad that I thought the pain could cause another psychotic break, and I increased my medication for a while. Looking back, I see the rejection was painful mostly because he had the self-esteem I wanted for myself. I somehow believed that I could achieve self-esteem through *association*. It is crystal clear now. That is not to diminish Tyler's attractiveness.

I was surprised when a fella approached me online who was in his twenties and had a thing for mature women. I agreed to meet him, and he said he was going to cook me a meal.

Immediately when I met him, I knew I was in trouble because he started kissing me in the courtyard of the apartment complex. I went inside and the kissing continued. I was very concerned with his sexual health, and since he had not had a STD test, I was somewhat eager to get him dealt with in a safe way. He was super sexy. I could have left, but instead I offered to give him a blow job with a condom. Before I even had time to get up from the bed, he was already hard again swinging it in front of me and celebrating his youth. I just excused myself and left.

I had hoped he would decide to have a HIV test and we could continue to see one another. He was enough to get my mind off Tyler. It was not to be. I experienced extreme anxiety over whether or not he had HIV, although he had assured me he didn't. In my anxious mind, I started thinking that perhaps I might have had a crack in my lips and that maybe if he had the virus I could have been exposed by kissing him.

I started thinking that I had to disclose to James what I had done because I didn't feel right taking chances with his health. I wrote James a text saying I had been with a man for a year who was HIV negative but had recently been with a fella in his twenties who had a thing for women my age, and although we had used protection, I did not know his HIV status. I said I did not want to put James' health at risk. I felt strongly about the morality of that.

When James got home from work, he was in a good mood, which made me wonder if he had read the text. So I asked him, and he said no and then started reading it. He started trembling and then asked if we could talk in the bedroom. He said to me that he wanted things just to be between us. I stated that I was not going to stop doing what I was doing.

He gave me a hug and said he had to go for a drive. I also went for a drive. Calvin knew what was going on.

While I was out, I got a call from Calvin saying to come home right away because James was trying to get Calvin to come out of the bathroom to talk. I said that I would be right home. When I got home, James was very angry and told me I had a week to get out. I now believe I had beat him at his own game.

20. Not the Only One Crazy

The nonsense started after this point. James was going after low hanging fruit in his antics with me. I was grateful to have Angelina. She was always patient and comforting to me. It was a few weeks before I could secure housing, and the time was difficult in the house. James was turning off the hot water, disabling the microwave, and hiding my blender that I made smoothies for the children with. He also took my tax documents, which I never recovered. He changed the Wi-Fi password so Calvin could not get on the Internet, but Amber and Mingus still had Wi-Fi. Calvin had school assignments requiring the Internet, but was not able to complete them.

Calvin got very sick with a strange rash. I asked James to pick up a thermometer when he was out, but he refused. That same night we were gone for most of the night at the ER, and when we got back at 4 a.m., both locks on the door were engaged; traditionally, we relied on one. James never asked about Calvin once, and he was sick for over fourteen days and saw four different doctors.

I had to have my keys on me continually because James was locking doors. I also slept with my phone under my pillow. Calvin had seasonal allergies one morning before school, and I asked James, with Calvin standing there, if Calvin could have allergy medication. James said, "No." I said, "There is some," and James said, "I don't care." James had the bedroom door locked, and I was forced to sleep on the couch. Also, my medication Breo for treatment-resistant asthma, which I was taking daily, went missing. I was smoking, at this point.

Then James started taking Amber and Mingus (age ten) away without saying anything to me. He also started trying to turn them against me by telling them things about me and my dating profile, which they started asking me about. He was also telling them he was going for sole custody.

I had a routine of snuggling with Mingus in the morning. Since I was now sleeping on the couch, the snuggle sessions were there. The sun was streaming in directly on Mingus' face one morning, so I went over to draw the blinds. James opened them up again. I said that I was closing the blinds so I could snuggle with my little man, and he said, "And I am opening them."

I tried to shield Mingus' face with a blanket, but it was not working, so I told him we would go downstairs to snuggle in his room. As soon as we headed down the stairs, James told Mingus he had to get ready for the bus. I told Mingus my phone said we still had ten minutes before the bus. Mingus related this back to James, and he said, "Well Mom's phone is wrong." I could see Mingus was confused but went to get ready for the bus as his father wanted him to.

Let me tell you about some other upsetting things James did in those days. Historically, I had a habit of getting into the children's candy stashes at Halloween and Easter, but I always confessed and replaced what I took or gave them extra money for my violations. I was always liberal with getting the children's favourite junk food if they ate their healthy food.

After one trip to James' parent's home, Amber and Mingus brought home some special cookies from their grandmother. I had noticed them and had no intention of eating them.

One morning, as the twins were having breakfast, James exclaimed, "Your cookies are gone!" I couldn't believe my ears. I didn't say a word, and Amber and Mingus didn't say a word. It was such an underhanded way to try and sabotage my relationship with them. I suspect he was trying to set me up to defend myself and have a showdown with my credibility in question because I had a history of getting into their candy

He took the twins away one weekend shortly before Calvin and I were due to move out. We spent the weekend moving our things left to me by my parents. We also took the cat "Lilly" that Calvin was extremely attached to, which turned out to be a smart move.

James came home earlier than he had told me he was going to come back, changed all the locks on the house, and told me by text. Calvin and I were not home at the time. I had been told by my lawyer not to move out before there was an interim child agreement for Mingus and Amber. I contacted the police. The police talked to James, and he reported he "feared for his safety," so I could not return. I even thought the police must be wondering, "What in the backwoods Florida swamps is going on here?"

If there was anything that could have made me sick around this time, it was the breakdown of the family and all the craziness. Stress is a variable for another psychotic break, and as I mentioned, the threshold is lower after the first break. Angelina talked to me more than once a day for support and thought that James was trying to precipitate another psychotic break for me so he could have sole custody.

My daughter, Amber, had a very hard time with the separation. I knew she was vulnerable because of the early years. She did not have a strong resilience inside her because of insufficient bonding. She needed a lot of support including a professional. I was relieved Mingus and Amber were twins and had the continuity of always being together going back and forth between separate households. Being developmentally matched and not antagonistic toward one another was also a good thing. With little on their side, I was searching for anything that might help.

Mingus had traditionally been closer to me, but James had turned him against me. Mingus was very critical of me, to my face, and challenged me on everything I said. Before Calvin and I secured housing, Mingus was saying things like, "Cheat on Dad once and you're done," "Did your lawyer talk to you about the things you removed from the house?" "I don't have to listen to you because this is Dad's house." (Children cannot think abstractly the way adults can. It is a natural tendency for them to see things or people as good or bad. It must be impossibly difficult for them to find any middle ground when they are already developmentally bound and being coached that one parent is bad). It took almost three years for me to recover some of the closeness that we once had.

Recently, I had a breakthrough from telling him I loved him, where he would simply reply "ok". He finally said back, "you too", delivered with a friendly wave. It made me melt.

In an effort to provide comfort for the children in my new three-bedroom home, I gave each child a furnished bedroom and decided that the front room couch would be my bed. (I call beds "nests" when speaking of them to the children, since it is a cute and cozy concept). I did not mind a bit and never felt like a martyr. I also bought three mattresses so we could camp out together in the front room until they felt more secure in their new surroundings.

James' lawyer challenged me on this sleeping arrangement, but my lawyer did research on the family bed and said as long as each child had a separate mattress it was fine. It has been three years, and we often sleep in the front room, "camp out style", with zero pressure from me. Calvin participates less and less, which is normal. I consider the front room like a therapy room. (Our sweet cat, Lilly, is always with us.) It is especially fun at Christmas sleeping next to the lit tree.

21. Doing What I Could

Calvin is very good to his younger siblings. He was nurtured properly, so he has an abundance of kindness and good will in his character. He is helping to make up for my failures, supporting them naturally without consciously trying. He is engaged and makes them laugh. Since he is still a teenager, he can relate to them in ways I can't. He takes pride in them and is protective. The twins and I are almost always in the front room, and they are always excited when Calvin joins. I have BBC Earth on in the background because it is a low stimulation channel. I like the children having an enriching exposure to science shows. I nicknamed Dr. Brian Cox "Smiley Billions" because he uses the word so often and radiates a bright happiness when teaching about the natural world and our universe. The only time I saw him look unhappy was in the G-force experiment. I believe it might have been at 4-G's when his happiness decayed. He strikes me as a poster person for high self-esteem. Calvin, Amber, and I are superfans of Sir David Attenbourough. JunsKitchen on Youtube is also a favourite. Jun's level of excellence is almost meditative to watch. He somehow pairs pristine cleanliness and cats in the kitchen as mutually inclusive. I imagine him being sought by Queen Elizabeth and Oprah (not at the same sitting, for now). The children hijack the TV for YouTube videos often, and it feels connected and close.

I try to negotiate with them on things so that they have a sense of power. I let them win often. I am quick to praise them for good social behaviour and their unique abilities. I rarely get angry, and I would say the home environment is supportive and pleasant with love between all. My twins rarely fight and they negotiate on one another's behalf if they think I need extra persuading. They adore Calvin, and they all love Lilly. I share 50% custody with James.

I am trying to create a happy home for my children. We share a lot of laughter, and I want the children to have an experience of a happy mother. The more children experience their parents as happy, the more they internalize the belief that they also have a right to be happy. As a side note, James had his ex-wife move into his house less than a few weeks after I moved out. It certainly confirmed my suspicion that he had not been faithful, beyond what I had known about, because the timing for his ex to move back in was so fast.

When I first moved out (2018), I was doing house cleaning for money. I had some difficult customers, but I was meticulous about cleaning and enjoyed it for a time. I had two people contact me, and it was like a cleaning test. When I arrived, the houses were perfectly clean. I feel they wanted someone to come in and say that. Believe me, I know what clean is. Like most eccentric people, I get hung up about garbage. For me, the thing is I take my garbage in my car every day and deposit it at one of several garbage cans in the community. I mostly target service stations, but I have found other ones. They are secret. Haha. I wonder if the garbage man and neighbours wonder why I only put recyclables out. They might wonder if the house is spilling over in garbage or any other number of things. I am going to say my day might be ruined if I can't take my garbage away from the house, but I am not sure. Lmao. (I am confident that any person crippled with OCD is going to benefit from this book.)

During those days I was continuing my self-study to become stronger, which I have detailed in upcoming sections. I was taking Olanzapine 2.5 mg. It was time to try and have a better hustle for money for an expensive surgery in California. Returning to nursing was out, with my history—not to mention, I would be required to take an 18-month refresher course to become licensed again. I barely got through the program the first time. I am an idea person, even if Calvin complains that I start talking about ideas with no context.

Calvin had a condition called gynecomastia and required uninsured cosmetic surgery. Gynecomastia is a condition where males have feminized breast tissue. Calvin was mortified by his condition. He would wear layers of clothes in the summer in an attempt to hide. He once described to me that he could barely walk because it was so distressing to him. He would never go in public places unless he absolutely had to. His confidence was zero. He had developmental challenges any teenager had to negotiate, but he was paralyzed by his gynecomastia. I thought if there was one thing I wanted to accomplish before I died it was to get him the surgery. Calvin was excited about going to California for the surgery, and humorously said we would get to meet all the people from GTA V. With my new work, I was able to financially achieve this surgery for Calvin in November 2019.

22. SOMETHING I DID WELL

I studied some excellent tutorial videos in May 2019 on how to give a good technical massage and started with my first client. I was advertising for providing mobile massages. I had found a job that was not going against my grain and where I could succeed. I had the funny thought I would compare quarterly earnings.

I very quickly learned that my clients were going to be mostly men, and they were looking for happy endings. My first client when I stepped into this territory was a bit cunning in that he encouraged me to continue massaging down low and seemed desperate for me to finish him so I jerked him.

I had some safety concerns and met a potential client who was easy to talk with. I will call him Lee. I was not looking to date. This gentleman was older than myself, but he was very kind and supportive. We kept meeting for coffee to discuss my concerns. He snuck up on me romantically.

It was a stroke of luck for me because he was a big fella who used to bounce at bars. Lee had knocked out an obnoxious person when he was seventeen, quit school, got a job the next day, and put himself through carpenter college. He built his first house when he was nineteen. He was not a fella to be messed with, but he showed a gentleness toward me, and I was vulnerable in this kind of work. By this point, I had encountered a couple clients who had made me feel threatened. I nicknamed one "Joudry Upstairs." I was afraid he was going to assault me. To get through to the end of the massage, I kept reminding myself of my dad's strength as a war veteran.

It was a bit comedic, but I told Lee in one conversation how I had an affair with a man for a year who women threw themselves at. Lee's response was, "He was the kind of man who women ran from and men too if they crossed him." He described himself as being unlucky in love. I liked that he wanted to protect me, and I thought it was sexy. I tend to project trust onto people, and he helped me see red flags I was not aware of. I am learning street smarts late in life. Here was a man who was the perfect combination of tough but sweet with me.

He was the divorced father of three children, but two had been killed tragically in two separate car accidents. I felt I was strong for having survived psychosis, but I felt like my strength paled compared to his. My respect for him allowed me to hear him in a way that I would not listen to others.

He dedicated himself to helping me screen contacts. He also encouraged me to hold onto my unique niche of not offering full service. I was feeling a lot of pressure, and had stepped into full service a couple times, but he kept telling me there was a middle market between the RMTs and full service providers, and I was a perfect fit.

Over time, I started feeling proud I was very unique in the limits I had. I started realizing the benefits to myself and my customers. One of the big benefits was assuring my own sexual clean health and my client's comfort and trust. I declined future high incentives for full service and companionship, as those are not a service that I offer.

I have also been approached by couples and people with fetishes, but I limit my exposure to that market. It was extremely hard for me to get into the mindset to even provide a half-assed attempt at humiliating someone. Really, I wanted to help him. When you see what I saw, not limited to drinking from a toilet, you would feel the same. I was very careful to screen clients to make sure they were of legal consensual age. I had a lot of hotel business from men traveling.

There is an escort and massage discussion forum, and I was reviewed there as providing an actual good topless massage with quiet, nice conversation and magic hands.

I would say that between 25 to 30% of the hits on my ad result in a booked massage. I have provided massage to clients traveling from Europe and coast to coast representing multiple ethnicities and varying social profiles. My clients range in age from twenties to eighty.

I sometimes worry that one of my oldest clients may end up coming and going at the same time. Some clients want some attention, and some are looking for good conversation, and most are interested in the overall experience. I had one client who told me that because sex is not on the table my massage is the only opportunity for him to enjoy pampering.

As with any business, there are challenges. The sex industry is a different world, for sure. In my first weeks, I was pretty naive. I used my actual name. I soon found out this was pretty dumb. I had a client call me who said since I provided my real name, to protect himself, he did a search on me. He said he found me on Facebook and found my father's obituary, and, therefore, knew my oldest son and ex-husband's names. He told me not to worry, but I can tell you I was freaking out. I came up with a work name, new email that day, and a burner phone shortly after with a new number. I still have a few clients who know my actual name from those days. I try not to offer personal information. I did slip and mention to someone I was writing a book, and then thought I better reassure him it wasn't an exposé.

Speaking of younger fellas... I had an appointment with one, and he told me he just loved milfs. It was my first appointment with him, and the appointment was going well. We made small talk for quite some time, and then I asked him who his favourite Kardashian was. I was thinking how pretty Kendall was. Without a moment of hesitation he said, "Kris!" It should not have caught me off guard, but it did.

I enjoy what I do, and people can feel this. That said, I have had to tone down my exuberance. This was necessary because clients were thinking I was their friend and some were looking for me to be their mistress. From a business point of view, over-familiarity is not good because clients tend to want more. I have addressed this by continuing to be warm and friendly but trying to keep the focus on them and creating a good experience for them. This is very much a balancing act because as Dale Carnegie says, some people go to the doctor to have an audience. People want visibility.

I have been offered soft and hard drugs, but I never accept. Some clients offer to pay me in medical grade marijuana. I don't use drugs, so that doesn't work. I have ended up at appointments where clients were under the influence. I had one client who had been drinking and put his hands around my neck. Luckily it was done in a more passionate way as opposed to threatening. I had another client who seemed like he was very horny and he couldn't stay still. When we were at the end, he was unable to maintain an erection and he said, "I might have had some coke this morning." To me it was just a little bit comical because he said "might."

Although I advertise "outcall only," I consistently get asked by clients about offering incall. There is a huge market for incall, and I mean huge. I do not offer incall because I don't operate a common bawdy house. There are big personal risks for a family offering incall. It is not lost on me that I am in a business of mostly attached males and cannot offer them a place to go. I have clients who promise discretion and respect if I can offer incall. I encourage them to rent a hotel room, but they often counter with a request for a car date. That is something I do not offer.

I had one client, a highly accomplished professional, who wanted to talk. He called it a consulting appointment. This gentleman had a serious drug smoking habit. He was using some type of glass tube and going back and forth from the kitchen to the table, where I was, every five to seven minutes. I naturally wanted to help him. After a couple consulting appointments, I joked with Angelina that if I couldn't help him I was going to give him *her* number and she could help him.

One client was particularly controlling in his approach with me. He said he needed a picture taken at the exact time he was texting me. He was concerned about discretion and told me to meet him in a nearby parking lot and for me to leave my phone in my car and go with him to his house in his car. My reaction was that I would meet him, but I would follow him in my car and would have my phone with me. It was a serious red flag that he wanted me to abandon my phone. He later tried contacting me from another number, but the scenario was the same, so I recognized it was him.

In terms of problematic clients, I do keep a log of their phone numbers so that I don't respond to them again. Experience has taught me, some ill-intentioned people can be quite slippery on a few levels. I remember a "triangle" model for assault from the days when I was with Charlie. The model suggests that assault happens when all three sides of a triangle are complete. The three sides of the triangle are represented by motivation, ability, and opportunity. I understand it is easy for these sides to be present in my business, so screening and Lee driving me to new appointments helps reduce all three sides. Siri is my best friend when I am with a new client. So far I have never had to say, "Hey Siri, call Lee." Lee has also shown me a few defensive moves. Lee has said if someone ever hurt me there is not a place on Earth they will be able to hide.

I had a couple clients whose body language suggested they were angry, although they did not act out. One fella who made that list met me at a hotel and had a very menacing laugh. He was talking to me about knives and how he had run over a cop, which landed him in jail, where he was praised for that act by other inmates.

I have one regular who seems to have a momentum-building countdown of several texts before the appointment happens. Because he curiously plays religious music in the matrimonial bedroom during these massages and is hyper-anxious about getting caught, I think it is risk that turns him on. He is very warm by text, but I haven't seen him eyeball-to-eyeball yet. It is a bit of a puzzle to me to figure out his psychology, especially the lack of eye contact. Maybe service providers offer the opportunity to act out a concupiscence struggle.

One client was very funny but did not intend to be. I went to his place to give him a massage. He had just come home from a family reunion at a lake. When I was at knee level, I discovered he was coated in coarse sand from the knees down. I made the observation and followed up with the suggestion that I not introduce that sand into the massage. He laughed.

I was once doing a massage for a client at one of his properties. Suddenly, there was a knock on the door. The knock became more insistent, and I was waiting for a reaction from him. He suddenly got up and said, "That is my wife, we have an open relationship." He started pacing and getting dressed. She was yelling at this point, and I was wondering if she was on board with the open relationship. He opened the door and addressed her outside. He came in and apologized and said we would continue another time. When I left, I was half waiting to get clobbered, but she was nowhere to be found. I have had some nasty phone calls from females.

One of my widowed clients had his sister call during a massage, and he said to her he was just sitting down to supper. When he hung up he said, "Another white lie." It struck me as funny.

My clients don't subscribe to "No Nut November."

Lee would be the person to step in and take my business phone if I was to have a second psychotic break. With psychosis being the wild card it is, I could do a lot of damage and invite a lot of trouble with my client list. I had a lot of clients who tipped their hat to Lee saying that they could not handle their girlfriend doing what I do. Part of what attracts me to him is that he can handle what I do.

As my ad evolved, I also was learning better tease techniques, and I had a client who gave me an education on deep testicular massage. This client showed me a video on Thai testical massage. I had always been careful around balls because males educate females on how mishandling can hurt, so I was always a bit cautious. The video I watched blew my mind as it was quite vigorous and was therefore the most surprising thing I have learned in some time. One version is in the supine position and the other is with the client on all fours. When I started using it, the results were great and that made me happy.

I was getting more and more hits on my ad, and occasionally one would clearly be a "recruiter." I was very afraid of them because the conviction rate for pimps is very low and trafficking is alive and well. I was warned about how all they need to do is get a "needle into you" and they have you. It took me a couple days to digest that story. Here is what I would like to offer them. "Tact is the ability to tell someone to go to hell in such a way that they look forward to the trip" (Winston Churchill).

I recently saw my very first client again. Since I saw him last he was the victim of someone who was psychotic. He sustained considerable injuries. We talked about it and he held no anger and was choosing to work toward his recovery instead of focusing on the assailant.

I was very impressed with his strength and shared that the body is always listening to our thoughts and he said he would remember that in his recovery.

A nerdy perspective is that orgasm is actually a reflex. A psychological arousal threshold has to be reached, with physical stimulation to trigger the physiological activation of the reflex. The exceptions that come to mind are a client who has been practicing release without touching and, of course, wet dreams.

Although I feel massage is within my ability range and something I am good at, I frequently find myself crossing over into psychology talks with clients when they seem receptive. Healing and psychology is a major drive and passion for me. I equally love the psychology behind romantic love. One of my regulars laughs with me about this tendency. I will never enter nursing again because I feel the scope of what I am about to share is beyond nursing, which is highly regulated. I want to help, and I don't want my hands tied. Based on this, I have begun a consulting practice to help people who have suffered more or less than I did. I have suffered very much in my past, but I am very happy, and I am so excited to show you the tools that are going to get you the big results. You have some invisible shackles, and I will help see them for the first time. Once you see them, you will quickly want to be rid of them. I will guide you with the best information my years of research has shown me.

The concepts to follow are mostly from Homer McDonald. He was in a league of his own. Homer and I had exhaustive conversations over the phone and I took lightning-speed jot notes. He said he was a detective working on my case. It is mostly from those notes that I am conveying the messages I want you to use. Homer passed away in 2016. My last conversation with him was in 2015. He was an incredible man, and I miss him. Homer was not wishy-washy about anything.

PART 2

"It's not your job to love me. It's mine."
—*Byron Katie*

Sometimes I will see an article on how to stand confidently or how to project one's voice or how to make eye contact or deal with rejection and many other ideas on behaving confidently. I want to assure you that so many of these things come automatically without thinking about them at all when you have high self-esteem. A person who enjoys high self-esteem and is happy is spontaneous, creative, quick to bounce back, and can easily find humor. There are so many things that flow naturally when you get the inside part right. I'm here to show you how to do it based on what helped me.

Since 2018, and through the separation and divorce, I have applied the help I received to finally feel happy and experience high self-esteem. The wheels came off but they went back on. I have resolute confidence in what works because I spent many years as a nurse in mental 'health', had so many problems, and have searched so hard for answers.

"We don't have the right to complain about something we're doing nothing about."
—*Homer McDonald*

Take a moment to score yourself on the following (where 10 represents excellent):

Please rate your overall level of happiness 1–10.

Please rate your level of self-esteem 1–10.

23. Happiness and Success

"No more postponing happiness."

Homer said, at a simplified level, happiness involves focus on what you can do, what you do have, and what you do like. Negative thinking is what you don't have, don't do, and don't like. The positive thinker gets more good things, and the negative thinker gets less and less. The person is either thinking poor me or lucky me. Intuitively, we all already know that feelings come from our thoughts. When we want to cheer someone up we say, "Think about good things." I am going to show you the "how."

Two kinds of happiness

1. Conditional—I will be happy as long as I'm getting my way.

2. Unconditional—I'm going to be perfectly happy whether I get my way or not.

HAPPINESS AND SUCCESS ANXIETY

Nathaniel Branden was the first person I knew of who addressed happiness anxiety. There is lots of content around it these days. I want to address the concept of happiness and success anxiety. I want to speak on this first, because if you are not comfortable with them, you may be driven to sabotage your efforts to feel better. Happiness/success anxiety will seek expression in our mood, the way we interpret other's behavior, our triggers, and pursuit of goals, just to name a few.

Happiness and success, for some people, create anxiety. This anxiety occurs in people who become nervous when things are going well. There are others who don't pursue their dreams. A little less obvious is the subconscious part, which can be seen in examples of self-sabotage. Happiness does not resonate with what they expect as natural for themselves. More often they wish for happiness, and it always seems to be something for the future (Branden, 1994).

I don't know anyone who doesn't identify with "wanting" to be happy, but for some it seems elusive. Happiness anxiety sets up residency in the subconscious mind for people if they have experienced early trauma or lived in an unhappy home growing up. Sandy Gallagher says "your own personal history of failure" can set you up to not go after your goals (Gallagher, 2018). This can lay the foundation for living an unhappy adult life by default. Sub-optimal has a certain familiarity to it. Sandy says that "the fear of going into uncharted territory of success can be more intimidating than fear of failure" (Gallagher, 2018). People can waste so much potential for good in their life with this happiness/success anxiety running in the background. Sometimes people will do the exact opposite to what they know is in their best interest.

Nathaniel Branden said to me people are more accepting toward their own good health compared to feeling happiness. He used the example that when people wake up in the morning feeling healthy, they think that is normal. He said when some people wake up in the morning feeling happy, they think there must be a mistake (Branden, 1994).

Understanding and acknowledging that the subconscious exerts an effect on our daily life is a step toward happiness, because you can reflect on your behaviors and knee jerk reactions and gain some conscious leverage. I think it is a good practice to address happiness /success anxiety through guided meditations specifically for happiness. The subconscious is much more powerful than most people are aware and can be charmed into producing good results.

Another way to harness the power of the subconscious is through visualization, the close cousin to meditation. This is a *huge secret weapon*. As we all know, professional athletes use this technique to improve performance. Visualization theory suggests that the subconscious mind handles visualization the same way it accepts reality such that it cannot set them apart (Maltz, 2015). The subconscious is an obliging companion and on duty 24/7. It was said that when John Cleese would have a creative problem he would hand it over to his subconscious by sleeping on it and often had the solution upon awakening. We can take inspiration from this and visualize to suit.

Your subconscious is always active, think about how your mouth waters either when your favourite food is in front of you or you imagine it. "When we visualize something we're priming ourselves to take action, we're telling our subconscious mind to figure out how to get the thing we're visualizing" (Hayden, 2018). When you have moments of insight and hunches, it is usually generated by the subconscious mind. I tend to have these moments in the shower or before sleep when I am relaxed. I sometimes wonder if my deep belief about what causes psychosis precipitated my psychotic break when those conditions were met.

....

"We look in the mirror and frown and then say,
'Oh my God the mirror is frowning back.'"
—Homer McDonald

....

Maltz (2015) explains we cannot achieve beyond our subconscious beliefs or self-image. If you see yourself as a depressed person, your subconscious will work in the background to bring reality into step with your self-image. Through visualizing ourselves achieving, we can start to change our vision of ourselves and what is possible. "Somehow before a person can change he must see himself in that role" (Maltz, 2015, p. 46). It is helpful, but not enough, to act in better ways. Visualization offers more impact than changing behavior alone, because the subconscious works hard to return what is planted. Please stretch to visualize yourself being the *ideal you* that you would be pleased with. Because we can't exactly 'outsmart' the subconscious, try the following. If you are experiencing resistance, you may begin with "what if…" as a way to make inroads. An example would be if you have difficulty imagining yourself owning the space you stand in, where you have historically tried to fade into the background. If it seems very hard to create the imagery of a bold version of yourself, begin this way. The more detail you can supply to your visualizations, the better, since there is more for your subconscious to grab hold of. You can imagine it like a story and play out the process of "becoming".

Day to day we behave and think in ways that reinforce our baseline experiences of happiness and success. Homer called it a happiness or unhappiness trap. We need to be one step ahead of the part of our mind that wants to be unhappy. He explained there is always a salesperson and a buyer in our internal dialogue. He said that we sell negativity in various ways and then say, "I'll buy," and then cry and complain.

"Everybody in the world is seeking happiness, and there is one sure way to find it. That is by controlling your thoughts. Happiness does not depend on outward conditions. It depends on inner conditions" (Carnegie, 1981, p. 71). Homer explains over and over that we never just have an event occurring. There is always a rational or irrational sales pitch. To illustrate, to me, that we are always dealing with the sales pitch in our head, he said the following:

"We are going for a walk and it starts to rain, but we are not dealing with the rain, we are dealing with the sales pitch.

I love the rain (no whining).
I hate the rain, and it is spoiling my walk (whining and very proud of my ability to hate).
Indifference about the rain, which is smart.

No situation is ever improved, let alone our feelings, by whining, crying, or screaming. We often believe these have the power to change things, but it is not true. When it comes to whining, crying, and screaming at others, it works the opposite of what we want because it creates pressure, which people on the receiving end react negatively to. We can do better.

T.D. Jakes, in his *Steps Video for Thought,* spiritually leads his congregation into the understanding that we grow in steps. "...All you have to do is stop complaining about where you are, because when you complain about where you are you do like Israel and you wander around in the wilderness because you are not eligible to make the promotion because you are grumbling about the level you are on right now. You are cancelling out the opportunity to go to the next level" (Jakes, 2014). He was explaining growth and trusting God to provide the next step as we learn to deal with opposition, conflict, criticism, and pressure on the step we currently occupy. He actually used the word 'rejoice' when speaking about these challenges.

HAPPINESS ANXIETY EXERCICE

Nathaniel Branden talked to me personally about the concept of happiness anxiety in 1998. I am going to share the exercises he used with me when I had one-on-one counseling with him by phone and in person. I did them daily for a long time. I encourage you to try to "unlock" your mind briefly and explore this idea.

Instructions Nathaniel gave me:

"I will provide you with a few incomplete sentences. Your job is to complete the sentences out loud, as quickly as you can. The freedom to answer with the first thought that comes to your mind is believed to be accessing some of your subconscious. Once insight is increased, changes in thoughts and behaviour may follow. (There are many customizable variations of this exercise to go deep into the subconscious.)

Answer each incomplete sentence with five to ten endings. (You can interchange the word "success" with "happiness.")

Happiness to me means...
If it turns out I have a right to be happy...
If my parents saw me living a happy life...
If my happiness could speak it would say...
One of the ways my happiness comes out is...

One of the scary things about being happy might be...
One of the good things about being happy is...
One of the bad things about being happy might be...
One of the ways I might sabotage my happiness might be...
It is beginning to dawn on me that..."
(Branden, 1998, Personal Interview).

If my mental illness could speak it might say...

HAPPINESS AND HUMOUR

"Nothing gives a person more comfort than a laugh."
—Homer McDonald

I want you to consider this. Homer McDonald told me, "Everything straightens up when we laugh." When we laugh, we lose our inferiority complex straight away. It is an interesting note that some of the funniest people have had great suffering in their lives. They instinctively realized that the way out of pain is through humour. Humour is always about pulling the rug out from under someone when they are not expecting it ("...and hope they don't come after you," as Tim, my Oreo friend said, *and wanted to be called Mr. Big in the book*). Laughing makes you feel superior and as if you have no problems. It puts you on top of any situation. Laughing also makes you feel friendly, confident, proud, and outgoing. I have always said, "Laughing is a type of being in heaven."

Please try this. I invented this little trick whereby I wake in the morning and set my "compass" on finding humour in the day. I can tell you, on the days I do this, it works, and I am able to find more laughs in the day.

HAPPINESS AND HEALTH

There is a feedback loop between happiness positively impacting our health and having good health helping toward our happiness. Oprah spoke with Deepak Chopra in one interview, and a very profound statement was made. He said, "Every cell in your body is eavesdropping on your internal dialogue" (Chopra, 2016). I thought this was tremendously important.

Further, we know that stress releases cortisol from the adrenal glands in the kidneys for the fight or flight response, which weakens the immune system. Trying to reduce your stress so that your immune system can be in peak condition for any virus or illness is worthwhile.

To develop the synergy between the subconscious and conscious mind so that they work toward the goal of happiness and health, I recommend meditation again. I am not an expert in the area, but I set my meditations on happy thoughts, images, and health. There are many excellent guided meditations on YouTube. My personal favourites are by The Honest Guys. If you are crunched for time, there are guided meditations for while you sleep. If you have trouble settling for sleep, these can be of double benefit as they guide you into sleep. Donald Hebb famously said that neurons that fire together wire together. It is believed the brain is somewhat plastic, so both meditation and better cognitive habits should become a better neural habit in the brain.

Occasionally, while meditating, I would have intrusive negative images, which I guessed had come up as a sabotage from my subconscious. Instead of resisting those, I would simply allow them to be there and give them space so they would dissolve and I could then gently bring my focus back to happy and healthy images.

Throughout the day, I would try to consciously focus on what I *do want* as opposed to what I *didn't want*. The purpose was twofold. First, focusing on what you don't want increases stress and fear. The second reason is the idea that if you are a race car driver and are focused on not hitting the wall, you are going to hit the wall. The energy we have available is better used seeking what we *want* as opposed to what we don't want.

In focusing on what you do want as opposed to what you don't want, I would encourage you to leverage the power of questions. The idea of "power" of questions came from fellow author Giulia Remondino in her book *Genius by Choice*. The mind wants to "solve," and presenting questions in terms of what you want as opposed to what you don't want will engage your natural curiosity and problem solving. This is an inherent part of how the mind works, and you can use that advantage.

Again, this comes back to the idea that every cell in your body is listening to your internal dialogue and organizing themselves through neurotransmitters and hormones to bring about that which you give your attention to.

With regard to our early experiences of happiness, the first years last forever, but learning is lifelong. The test for when learning has occurred is generally when behaviour changes. Behaviour could be represented by a new pattern of self-talk, behaviours, and feelings.

A tripping point to consider is that of habit. It is true that we have habitual patterns of thinking and they are a path of least resistance. In this book, I am asking you to interrupt and stop these patterns of thinking because they are self-perpetuating. Tony Robbins' information says that when new knowledge comes up against *patterns*, it is usually the patterns that win (Robbins, 2018). Try to remember this as a potential obstacle and recognize it may keep you stuck if you are not willing to work at better and new patterns. Be intentional with applying the ideas in this book and let yourself "feel" what it will be like to get the results you want. Emotional involvement with learning creates more anchoring of learned material. It is a kind of cognitive glue. This is *inspired* learning. If you ever watch anything on Tony Robbins, you will see this in action as he emotionally involves clients.

24. SELF-ESTEEM

Our personality interacts with our primary figures of attachment and broader experiences, and helps to shape our self-concept. There are certainly people who are naturally confident at a young age and carry that through their adulthood. Many other people suffer with low self-esteem. Self-esteem as defined by Nathaniel Branden is "the experience that we are competent to cope with the basic challenges of life and we are worthy of happiness" (Branden, 1994, p. 20). Branden is very specific on what is involved in achieving self-esteem. He also coined the term pseudo self-esteem. My experience linking my self-esteem to whether I was able to satisfy Branden's six pillars criteria resulted in increased anxiety for me. You will see in the discussion of praising oneself that a person's self-esteem can be high without all the measuring. I believe Branden was brilliant on many ideas and, for me, especially the happiness piece. He offered modern psychology many valuable insights. I really liked his book *The Disowned Self*. In my experience, self-esteem is fluid but absolutely within reach. Self-esteem has a tremendous reach in your enjoyment of life. It can greatly be improved if one knows how.

Self-esteem and confidence are somewhat-related in terms of how we experience ourselves and those around us. To set them apart, I will use the example that I am not confident about my math ability. I am in a good relationship with reality and I have never been smart about math. My acceptance of this has nothing to do with my good feelings about myself. We cannot all be confident in all tasks.

My self-esteem is rooted in my acceptance of myself, my shortcomings, and my areas of strengths. I embrace them all and carry no shame as a result of counseling with Homer. I will talk later about shame. If you have self-acceptance and praise yourself for all that you are, you won't look for feelings of self-worth in social media likes, bank accounts, or appearance. The argument is lost the minute you believe you need to prove your worth. Many people falsely believe the love of someone else will supply self-esteem. I made the mistake believing it could be achieved 'by association' with someone who had it. Self-esteem is an inside job or you don't have it.

A person who loves themselves does not think others are "less". A person with high self-esteem may recognize low self-esteem in another person. This has absolutely nothing to do with a person's *worth*. Melanie Yates delivered this so succinctly in her book *Happy, Joyous, and Free*. It must be shared in her words: "...You can never increase or decrease your worth. You can't lose it and you can't find it. Your worth is a set point in the universe. You have no control over it" (Yates, 2020, p. 26).

Calvin showed me a YouTube video called "Pimp my Wheelchair" (Miller, 2016). The gentleman featured in the video had cerebral palsy, and I can tell you he had more *game* than many people I have met. Not a drop of self-pity.

A cute aside: Mingus has his own phone. He has a condition called Goldenhar Syndrome. He doesn't have any shame about only having one ear. One day a telemarketer called him. He stayed on the phone for a long time with her. At one point he said, "I don't know what you are talking about!" Then she was trying to get the adult of the house on the phone and he said, "You called my number!" Then I heard her ask him if he was nineteen years old and he said, "No." She was becoming exasperated at this point, and Mingus said, "I can't hear you, I've only got one ear." It was pretty funny.

Although it is human nature to compare, good self-esteem is an internal experience and not comparative (Branden, 1994). That said, human beings are hardwired from an evolutionary perspective to make judgements/comparisons. Our survival depends on the actions we take from judgements/comparisons about what is good for us or bad for us. We cannot and should not try to extinguish this. I just wanted to move your thoughts in the direction that having good self-esteem liberates you from some of that comparison between yourself and others. In case you are thinking I have written a book on self-esteem and this is all I am offering, let me reassure you I am just setting the table. The answers are found in the collection of topics to follow. The finale of its attainment is in learning how to praise yourself.

25. Needs and Wants

*"There's only one thing that's better than getting what you want:
it's to know that you can be happy whether you get it or not"*
—Adyashanti

We want to get out of pain. Pain has no intrinsic value other than temporary teaching. We don't want any permanence to pain. Homer explained to me the easiest way to get ourselves out of pain is with regards to *wants* and *needs*. This means to enjoy things but don't feel self-critical if you don't have them. A practical example, "When you go to the dance, you will approach women, and you will not care if they say yes or no." People's tendency is to take a *want* and exaggerate it to a *need*. A person is thinking if I prefer x I must have x. If I prefer something, "I need it and I must have it" causes anxiety. For example, approval is nice, but we don't actually need it. Reality is not the problem. The problem is always calling a preference a need. I must have what I prefer. Society says there is no preference, it is a need. Oftentimes, PhD's and psychologists have the same philosophy, saying you need what you want.

There is a consequence that shows up psychologically when preferences get elevated to needs. Need always comes with pressure and anxiety. We are exerting pressure on ourselves, others, and sometimes on the environment. The weaker a person's desire, the more likely they will get it. Most people believe the stronger your desire the better, and you just work your ass off. Homer used the example of a man not getting as much sex as he wants. The way a man fucks up his sex life is wanting more, wanting more. Since something is nice, people become desperate for more, and that is a mistake. The man thinks, "I sure do desire sex, and if I want it I must get it." In this way, he pushes sex away from himself. Caring too much pushes away the thing you want. If the man would say, "It would be nice, but it is only a preference, and I can be happy without it," it would encourage his partner to feel warmer and friendlier.

People don't see anything wrong with "needing." If we are needing what is not already in existence, we increase stress and frustration for ourselves and often get less. We become critical of ourselves because we have not achieved what we wanted. The man who strongly desires to get a promotion doesn't get one. The man who is content gets the promotion.

Homer said to me "God is sadistic." He wants to give you the opposite of what you want, it's where he gets his jollies. He will give you an overweight body. You say you want to save the marriage—you will not get what you want. You can fool God—if God thinks you are excited about being single again, he will save your marriage. You have to be dedicated— you have to fool your kids, the pastor, everybody. Every breath you take, you are excited about being a single woman. The husband will change his mind and want to save the marriage. (I interpreted him to be saying God is going to show you you don't need what you think you need. Homer presented concepts to have maximum impact).

A clue that I can't tolerate not having my own way is represented in the following statements... "If I don't like it, it shouldn't be," or "Oh my God this is a big deal, how can this be happening to me?" If I say, "I don't like it and that's perfectly ok," I am loving reality. I am a big girl, and I can accept something I don't like. So, when we believe in preferences, we feel secure, and the environment is more likely to respond favourably. Homer used the example of a person who was told by the doctor that he was going to die within a year. He was thinking, "I prefer to live so I must live." Then he decided, "I have a year to live so why not have some fun?" He starts having fun doing his hobbies, and he forgets about his symptoms, and his symptoms get better. He's not thinking about dying anymore. He changed "I must live" to "it is just a preference," that's all it is.

Another example is a policy of needing people to like you. It is not hard to imagine this anxiety because we have all felt some degree of it. That pressuring attitude causes us to make social blunders. For example, we will lack the natural spontaneity of conversation and humor. Understanding we don't need others to like us relaxes us so we are more comfortable in our skin. You get something if you prefer it. If you need it, you destroy it. If I prefer something, it may be a practical problem but not an emotional one.

Homer said when you believe in needs, you believe in insecurity. Boiled down further, it is an addiction to guilt, and self-pity follows. It starts with some kind of frustration, something I want and I am not getting. I want my child to always be smiling, but my child is crying, so I hit myself over the head with a stick (my standards). I say, "Bad me, shame on me. If I was smarter, this wouldn't be happening." "If I was a better parent, my child would be laughing." As a result of hitting myself over the head, I cry with *poor me*, and I feel depressed.

It is hard to see guilt as a problem when everybody thinks it is smart. For example, I should feel guilty if my performance is inferior or I am not attractive enough. I want to jump up and down and criticize myself. I can stop that.

There are two words that explain all human behavior according to Homer. These words are "smart" and "stupid." A person is upset for one reason. They think it is smart to be concerned and think it would be stupid not to be concerned. All thinking has to have an aura of dignity.

Believing in *shoulds* and guilt hurts our happiness. Homer kept pounding the following into my head. We think it is smart and virtuous to hit ourselves over the head with guilt. After we hit ourselves over the head with the hammer called guilt, that is dressed up in ribbons because we attach virtue to it and we cry in pain, self-pity, and depression. Conventional wisdom says guilt is the voice that gets us back on track, but when we sober up, we see guilt does not do this. Guilt is the cause of self-pity. You can see the pattern if you examine instances where you gave yourself a hard time for something and judged yourself on trying to live up to a standard. The harsher the judgement, the more guilt is experienced followed by self-pity and depression. For example, "I failed to save enough money for Christmas presents for my children, I am a bad parent." The person in this example goes quickly from guilt to self-pity and depression.

Homer told me about a client of his who lost his job at the bowling alley because, in his words, he was masturbating many times a day. He was also going to see a priest. Homer told him, "I want you to masturbate every time you want to and is possible." That is going to make this advice very different and a great thing. The client reported back to Homer later that the last time he had masturbated was a few days ago. Guilt was the problem, not masturbating.

Homer said that the habit of feeling guilty prevents us from considering other options. For example, I should feel guilty and like a failure if my husband leaves me... no other choice. Instead, "I'm so glad my marriage is failing, I'm so proud of myself." If my marriage is failing and I think I would be stupid to call myself smart and a success and get out of it, I don't give myself that option. I can't go through a doorway to Heaven over this doorway that says Hell.

Homer explained to me that self-pity is a spin off from guilt. Self-pity comes from "bad me, stupid me" blaming the frustration. It's not the frustration, it's me selling guilt. You can't cure something while believing in the cause of it. Once you understand it is not smart to suffer, guilt loses its credibility. All that is needed is a touch of learning, and then we are moving on.

Society says you've got to have desire for what you don't have because you wouldn't be motivated. To handle this objection, consider that you would be motivated by pleasure and love. We always perform better when we feel better. "I'm so glad and proud that I want to do even better!" People believe that desiring what you don't have is essential and good. Homer says that desiring works against things being better and instead pushes things away. My interpretation is especially when it comes to getting what we want from other people as desiring comes with pressure. For example, having a strong desire to make a good impression, you don't. The other distinction would be whether there was "whining" about the *desiring more* or "confidence" about the *desiring more*. Desiring to perform better in sports is likely coming from a place of confidence and determination versus whining.

Needs and Wants

Our emotions come from our sales pitch inside our heads. If we are unhappy, we are selling ourselves on unhappy thoughts. Fatigue is always an essential part of depression. The reason a person is feeling fatigued and depressed is because they have been practicing a lot of negative thinking. If you try to understand why you feel this way, you will continue to feel that way. This is because you continue to reinforce negative neural pathways. It is the "habit" of how our brains work. The more you walk a path in the woods, the more the earth is pounded down and it is hard to deviate from it. Another example is, when I ask you not to think about the word "apple," it is "apple" that you are thinking about. We want to displace the negative by focusing on the positive, and the most effective way to displace the negative is to not give it a constant supply of energy. Examining negative feelings is not an effective method to experience better feelings. If you try to understand, try to analyze, and put meaning behind your suffering, you've already added your own interpretation, so you lose objectivity right away.

We can see our neediness show up in our temper. My temper comes from my thinking, whining, and screaming that things should go my way, believing it is smart to be upset and the opposite would be stupid. Society has taught us to be crybabies. All problems come from adding to reality. If I don't like it, it shouldn't be. Homer said temper is ridiculous, "I can't be happy unless I get my way." Nobody knows how to spell "some" meaning we want things exactly the way we think to be ideal. I can be happy while not getting my own way. Through preferring instead of needing. "It would be nice," A willingness for the negative to happen.

Another way we can look at this was described by Homer, whereby needing things to be a certain way means we hate when things are not up to our standards. Hating also results from taking a preference and calling it a must have. This is conditional happiness. The hating is the whining and crying, and the meaning of hating causes stress. We are proud of our ability to hate. People believe if they hate something it somehow has power to stop that which they do not like. Something happens I don't like so I bang my fist on the table demanding God do it my way. God says no. Next time prefer something be different, but it's ok if it's not and therefore not throwing a tantrum. Sometimes I wonder if wealth doesn't handle this for many people. In one sense, wealth keeps people comfortable so that everything can go their way, which may be it's ultimate appeal. I wonder if that resonates as truth for you?

The main idea I am excited for you to grasp, and I had to grasp, is the difference between taking a want and calling it a need. It is a procedure to help anybody in any kind of situation. If we can understand that most of the things we say we need are simply wants, we are immediately more relaxed and happy. We can identify that and see our problem is only imagination. This is one of the most powerful ways to reduce anxiety in ourselves. This will, in turn, drive up our levels of creativity and playfulness, and ironically we will be more likely to achieve our wants.

Homer cited Byron Katie who wrote *Loving What Is* saying hating is the attachment piece. In other words, we are attached to needing reality to conform to our wishes and hate reality if it is not to our liking. He said Katie basically teaches when you think about something you have stress or affection. If you have affection, you don't have any stress.

Homer said we can't "let go" when we hate. An example would be, I hate it when my partner is late so I can't let go of *needing him to change that behavior*. There is one distinction that is necessary to mention. Homer said that acceptance does not mean we cannot do anything. It does not mean *no action* or continuing to endure. You can respect your dislike and translate it into action. In the example of my partner being late, instead of whining and pressuring him to change, I can decide to go out by myself and have a good time on my own or decline a date night next time so that my time is not disrespected. "I'm fed up with this kind of treatment, so I am getting on with life." We don't have to waste futile energy and time trying to change someone else when they are simply being themselves. This establishes healthy boundaries. The other benefit is it brings us closer to a place of forgiveness.

When a person says they hate something, they are under stress, which has a negative effect on the body and the environment/situation. Hating always comes from taking a preference and calling it a must have. For example, I hate it that I can't memorize better. I pressure myself when I demand of myself that I memorize better. I am better served by *preferring* better memorization and strategize accordingly.

I was rejected by others after my psychosis, and Homer and I talked about friends. He said we are brainwashed. "We should" whine or "have to whine" if people don't like us and don't see we have the freedom to be happy. He said in these circumstances, the sales pitch reads, "Can't be happy, and it would be stupid to not want friends." He said if I prefer something, then I am just having fun doing things that move me toward x. For example, instead of *needing* friends, I can learn to be very happy without them. He said friends are not pure gain as they often want favours and so forth. This peace of mind makes me more attractive, so by being at peace over rejection, I am more likely to gain friends. He said, "Achieve something by reducing the importance of it." "I like being friendly" is not me seeking friends. He said it is good to be rejected by people as it will make me stronger and gives me a lot of freedom. If I don't care whether the other person is a friend or not, I have freedom from anxiety. I don't need to measure my worth in this way. It is not true that I cannot like myself until someone else likes me. "I want people to criticize me if they want to." He said your subconscious will instantly argue against this, saying it is crazy. The habit of fearing criticism will fight for it's life. "I am so fragile, I can't ever be criticized, I can't stand it." Instead of saying, "How dare that person insult me," practice saying "I'm glad she said that." It is not important to be worshipped by everybody. I don't have to change my position or contort myself to fit into a certain box just because someone criticizes me. If you have the attitude that you don't need any friends, gradually people want to be friends because you have the peace of mind that they want.

Standards play a big role in our happiness. Standards are not inherently wrong, but when they are used by us to make ourselves feel bad, it is a misuse of standards. They are fine if they are helping, but when we are complaining because we are not measuring up, they are harmful. We want to use them in a constructive way.

Society says you've got to believe in shoulds and should nots. The standards are "I should, we should". Instead of "I should aim to be a perfect mother," try, "I love being an imperfect mother." A belief in standards where you are criticizing yourself is not good. Brag on yourself and pat yourself on the back. "I could be doing worse but I'm not." Homer said we have a hammer disguised as a bunch of flowers, but I don't see it as a hammer. All I see are the beautiful flowers. But if they are only flowers, why do I have pain from the hammer blow? This hammer is not flowers...it's a hammer, and I'm not going to hit myself on the head with it. Most people's religion is believing in shoulds, and they fuck their happiness. It's the opposite of what everybody thinks; we don't *need* to succeed. "Must do well, must be loved, or believe it is smart to feel deprived if we're not getting everything from our mate" are all supporting self-pity. You can employ standards in a calm and matter of fact way. For example, it is desirable to be on time. I can have a standard of acting cheerful and friendly—not as an excuse to make me upset if I don't measure up. I would like to do well. I can only do my best. Personally, I have high standards of cleanliness, so I dive into cleaning and feel good. It doesn't cause me pain. The following are examples of pain associated with needing things to be a certain way.

"I don't want..."
"I don't like..."
"I can't stand..."
"If he loved me enough, he would..." (sales pitch for pain)

These are examples of needing and whining. It is never the situation but the whining. The essence of mental disturbance is blaming the situation. The whining kind of anger is passive and blaming. "He shouldn't be upset with me, I don't deserve that." Or "It is so terrible that I have physical pain." Physical symptoms are never the problem; common sense dictates medication and rest. Whining wants to keep going and calls itself standards.

26. Giving Up Worry

"Worry is a product of using your imagination poorly. If you are going to future-trip, go to a desirable destination. You're making it up anyway, so make it something you would actually want."
—Aimee Allen

The next issue we visited was worry. Judgements about ourselves as parents are rampant. Parents spend enormous amounts of energy worrying. Society has taught us to always be in some state of anxiety. The apparent belief would be that worry was protecting me. I had a tremendous amount of self-criticism, worry, and guilt over not being able to nurture my twins as much as my first born. We have been brainwashed that worry is an *intelligent* and *loving* thing to do and everybody is doing it. The other belief is you don't care if you don't worry. This makes the pain defensible and worry a virtue. This is another example of behavior being driven by what we consider to be smart or stupid. You can't get rid of something while you are arguing for it and calling it a virtue. You've got to change the argument.

Worry carries a mask of dignity about it. "I just wish my daughter would quit smoking"— that's just banging my head against a brick wall. Love and happiness claim good work. Worry actually slows down good work. Homer said worry and self-pity are twins. Self-pity says bad things are happening now. Worry is future oriented. Both talk about what we don't want, don't have, and can't get. Fear says, "I am your friend and want to protect you." Homer says, "No, fear is what we need protection from." You don't need to worship your fear. You can examine the threat and take what action is available to you instead of passively feeling worry. We make a decision to act and then the worry is gone. A touch of common sense and good judgement gets you out of the road when a car is coming. We are brainwashed that we should worry and whine and don't have the freedom to be happy. Don't kiss the ass of worry and fear. Children take the pain of fear and turn it into a game, a pleasure, like going to see a scary movie.

We see the bear and run instinctively. Worry is like a forty-pound weight around most people's neck, but we feel virtuous about these weights, beautifully packaged.

Homer chastised me to snap me into reality on this subject. He said, "This is so good for your children to have a worried mother." Worry advertises itself as love; it is an excellent salesperson. "How lucky can a woman be, I get to worry all the time." He said worry is one of the most popular hobbies. "I am so worried" is whining. Worrying is a bad habit and everybody is doing it, "Count me in." I have been doing it all my life, and my mother did it too. "I'm so worried" has to have an aura of dignity about it. Everybody gives it dignity. Worry does not want to die. Whining and worry will never run out of excuses. Whining and worry are excellent salespeople.

In my mind, I was thinking I was a poor mother and thinking I should be a better mother and should have spent more time with the children. Homer said I was not aware that this was a big fat mistake. He said when I hold the thought, "I should have been a better mother," it gives me guilt, stress, fatigue, and pressure and makes me a worse mother now. The truth is I should have been a partially invested mother because that is what I really wanted at that time. He told me I was having fun putting on a show about how guilty I was. There were reasons I was not more involved at the time. Today I would do a better job parenting very young children because I am not in pain psychologically. There is no value to feeling guilty about my past shortcomings.

Instead of worry and guilt over my past failings, I would be better off being comfortable with the reality I did an inferior job parenting in those days. He said, "Focus on now and whether you're giving them a healthy vision of happiness." How kids turn out depends on how not to make a big deal out of stuff, forgive, and forget. Show them a vision of happiness and show pride in them. **Homer told me being a better parent is not the goal. Stop whining is the goal.** The goal is a happy tone of voice about whatever is going on. "I'm an imperfect mother, I love it, I am human." This makes me a more relaxed and happier mother for my children. In her book, *The Power of Human Energy*, Renata Francetić explained that children pay attention to the energy of their attachment figures. She asserted that they feel the energy around them and internalize it, especially as language is still developing.

Society has brainwashed us to feel guilty every single breath, from kids to work. If other parents or colleagues are better than us, we can enjoy that. We have believed we did not have a choice but to feel bad. We have been trapped into being bothered if others are superior. It is only a bother to me if I whine about it. The most important thing in our lives for our children, and by example, is our emotions. *If we are happy, we, and they, have it made.*

I can remember discussing my exploding on Calvin with Homer. (It was not abusive, but I was feeling guilty.) Homer counseled me to say, "It was a mistake. There is no reason I should be perfect." There is no room for "A mother should, a mother should." He reminded me I am not going to have perfect control over my child. Don't throw a tantrum over it, just prefer. He told me to prefer I behave better in the future, but it is ok to not have what I prefer. I prefer that next time I not over-react, but if I do, I will forgive myself. The secret condemning happens over needing control over my child. I "prefer" to have control and that is enough. He encouraged me to be happy with Calvin the way he is and to stop worrying. This is not to suggest we don't have rules or expectations for our children. For example, Calvin is a bit of a dreamer, and I will not impose my ambitions on him, but I do have expectations that he will keep his room clean if he wants to go driving with my car.

It was funny. When I was teaching Calvin to drive, I wanted him to slow down over railway tracks, so I said, "Up on the gas," which he interpreted as "step on it." One night, Calvin and I were out driving and the headlights were dim. I mentioned it seemed like we were driving by candlelight.

I like my children to eat healthy foods, and I have to rein in my neediness over this. The classic workaround is to give them any junk food they want, providing they eat the healthy items. I have jokingly threatened Calvin that I am going to put him back on infant formula if he doesn't eat better.

I tell Mingus a little story called "Fear the Bully" to help him deal with his fears. Since children respond well to challenges, I frame it as such. I told Mingus fear gets its kicks out of scaring people. Fear wants to get bigger and bigger and make Mingus smaller and smaller so Mingus is afraid to do things. I told Mingus the way to win with fear is to give fear affection and welcome it. This takes away fear's power, and fear will stop coming around so much. The first time I told this to Mingus his eyes were wide with wonder.

27. CONTROLLING THE TONE OF YOUR VOICE

"We mistakenly believe that whining gets... but instead a happy voice, and face, gets money, a trim body, and sex"
—Homer McDonald

Beyond understanding the distinction between needs and wants, there is another way you can move yourself into greater relaxation and happiness. When there are circumstances we cannot change, we actually have another option. An opportunity exists for you to control the tone of your voice in your head and create positive feelings. Homer says when we are unhappy we are always using a whining tone of voice in our head. He says to state the negative in a calm soothing tone of voice. "Yesterday I made a fool of myself in public and it's perfectly ok, I am human." This gets us off the hook for feeling bad and gives us power to feel better quickly.

Every thought we have we are painting it with a colour... tone of voice. We form a habit of whining. (1) I've been doing it all my life. (2) Everybody else is doing it. (3) There is always a sales pitch or a story that dignifies the whining, and it gives me a (4) self-righteous feeling. "I don't want" in a whining voice is another excuse for poor me. Whining that I don't have a friend and everybody has a friend, for example. This protects my thinking that I am deprived. He says whining will argue it has good reasons. We can change the tone of voice in our head to joy or humour. Our joyful tone is under our control. We're the boss of our tone of voice in our head. We can get to the positive feelings very quickly by changing the tone of our voice. Homer said that years ago a doctor he admired simply said that if you change the tone of voice the meaning changes. The formula is to state the negative and admit it in a calm soothing tone of voice.

We can practice travelling the bridge between the negative and positive feeling by adding a positive tone of voice about reality. What might otherwise take days can occur in minutes. The tone of joy cancels out hurt and anxiety. **I control my future by my tone of voice;** we do better when we feel better. A happy tone in your thinking supplies energy and motivation to get better results.

Problem tone of voice: whining, screaming, crying
Good tone of voice: soothing, reassuring, joyful

Here are examples:

"I look forward to him being mad. I want him to be angry because he likes it..."
"I'm so glad I am inferior..." (say it like I won a medal)
"I am so glad I am shy..."
"I'm on the short end of the stick, but I love it..."
"I am so glad my husband is boring..."
"Divorce, I can do that. You name it!..."
"I love my overweight body..."
"My husband is leaving me. I'll find someone else or be happy alone..."
"I'm having a rough day, excellent, excellent..." (word excellent implies self-approval and joy)

You can practice this with energy and a lilt in your voice. Your old habit is going to argue, "That's not me," or the part of your mind that says, "But you don't understand." Be willing to experiment with this new idea. Homer says there is a constant sales pitch going on in your mind night and day of why you should not be happy. We're always in inner conflict. On one hand, we want to get rid of pain, but we also argue for worry, guilt, and self-criticism. Lots of times the part of your mind that wants to be unhappy outsmarts the part that wants to be happy. I defend the whining saying it shows I have brains, it's smart to whine, and everyone else is doing it. We argue there are certain circumstances where whining is warranted such as if kids are unhappy or husband is leaving. I would be stupid if I didn't whine under these conditions. He says people will say it is "crazy" to love it when your mate gets upset. He says that which *looks* crazy is actually sanity because it can be argued that the person who is loving reality and *not in pain* is actually the one who is not crazy. Homer was not the only person to address this. Marcus Pierre Bowen Jr. said the following: "There are drugs we are taking that we don't even realise we are consuming" (Bowen, 2020, p. 31). In his book, *Surviving the Unthinkable*, he describes complaining as a destructive drug that some people are addicted to.

Further, the more we hate others getting upset, the more it encourages them to be upset. Homer underscores that hating is the only problem and that a person either believes in hating or they believe in happiness.

Homer liked Byron Katie, and he said she talks a lot about being at peace with things as they are. Homer departed from her teaching and said there is nothing wrong with *wanting* something, but there is a difference between whining or saying it with confidence. There is no problem with wanting things as long as we are not whining about it and saying it with confidence. An example is the man who says with confidence that he *wants* a woman or "nothing is going to stop me, nothing is going to interfere." (To be clear, this does not mean disrespecting boundaries). There is a difference between "I should be doing better" (whining) versus "I want to do better." "I can" and "I will" are not whining either.

Homer furthers his idea and says it is the whining tone in our voice that carries the pain. He says we whine in our head about how things are. He encourages, as an example, to say cheerfully in one's head, "I am so glad they are critical of me, they are feeling self-righteous and that is perfectly ok." I gently present this idea to Amber when she feels criticized about her gender identity so she will not feel "less" and identify with being a victim. I also remind her that kids who are condemning are looking for a way to feel powerful, and putting others down is not a healthy way to feel powerful. Looking for power is one of the ways bullies operate. True personal power comes from knowing how to operate one's mind. That said, Homer maintained that accepting does not mean zero action. Amber is free to talk back or report the person, as she wishes, if someone is bullying her. The very most important item is that she consciously frames the bullying as a poor power maneuver, and, secondly, rejects it. The subconscious mind is impressionable, and part of the way we protect it is by consciously rejecting and reframing incoming information.

The other approach to interrupt the whining is anger. You can do this by saying to yourself, "Shut up." Homer says the healthy type of anger has some excitement to it, getting angry at the self-pity. This application is authoritative, simple, and powerful as fuck. (Homer used the word "fuck" pretty often to stimulate me to wake up.) He says anger kills the fear. He said to imagine myself in a boxing match. If I am focused on what he is going to do to me, I am in pain. If I am focused on what I am going to do to him, there is no pain because I am not passive.

Impotent anger—whining, stuck
Potent anger—growling or barking, stimulus for action

You can also ridicule the whining. "There I go whining again, isn't that funny!"

Homer cited Victor Frankel's book *Man's Search for Meaning* from the 40s where Frankel talked about paradoxical intention. Homer said Byron Katie was not the first to discover the turnaround. He said a doctor who was troubled by sweating said to himself, "Today I sweat a pint, tomorrow I will sweat a quart." You can't fear what you are wanting. Most people would say "You can't be happy about being nervous!" Excited about being nervous... dismissed as crazy.

As I mentioned in my introduction, I do not believe in black and white, but, rather, grey. Many of us would love to find an algorithm or flowchart to life with guarantees and no risk. There are no absolute prescriptives. We are not machines. I would never, for example, think that someone should *skip* over the five stages of grief identified by Kübler-Ross. That said, I am aware there are end-of-life celebrations that focus on positives. I like to look to nature for some objectivity. We can look to nature to see evidence of sentient animals grieving. Elephant families visit the bones of their deceased and caress them with their trunks. We know dogs mourn. I saw on BBC Earth a whale cow supporting her deceased calf for weeks before surrendering it to the depths of the ocean.

In my late teens, when I was studying Desmond Morris, he talked about humans being the ape that weeps. He essentially said this is a social evolutionary design that signals others and solicits compassion. Don't ask me to reference it, as I don't currently have any of his books. I just never forgot it.

If someone asked me what the biggest distinction is between humans and other great apes, I would have a number of thoughts. It's certainly not the use of tools. We have seen fish on BBC Earth that use rocks they pick up in their mouths to crack open crustaceans. It is not playfulness; offspring in many predators learn to hunt through play. Play also strengthens social bonds. Prey species also play. It is not a 'sense of self'. Mirror studies were convincing before the final test where the ape's hair was dusted, if I remember correctly. The ape used the mirror to identify the difference and removed the dust. It is not language potential, either. Koko the gorilla communicated in sign language that she wanted a baby, and when she was given a companion, she signed, "Wrong, old". So Koko even had some imagination. (Higher primates should have some evaluative insight that allows them to exploit opportunities around resources and regulate some of their behavior.) It's not even altruistic behavior. I remember a book called *Good Natured* by Frans de Waal I read in my 20s that showed apes compensating and caring for another ape. In the world between my ears, I wonder if some higher animal species can enjoy some measure of humor. Humor correlates with playfulness. If humor is the difference between expectation and results, surprise may be enjoyed on a continuum. Humans enjoy the full expression, with laughter.

The biggest difference I see is **our ability to edit our mind** through the application of our imagination, paired with intention, which *assumes insight*. But, because I like to test things for validity within the limits of my mind, I already identify a limitation. From my experience in the sex industry, I am going to say that kinks are not able to be rewritten, even though they are often supported by feelings of shame, which *is* treatable. I believe when fetishes form during psychosexual development, it is more akin to 'imprinting' with an extended, but limited, window. Imprinting is permanent, so after the window closes it is essentially hardwired. Now you can interpret this limit as disappointing, because I am highlighting areas of weakness in my position for influencing our minds, or you can take it as a sign I test everything. Therefore, what I do advocate, I believe. (Not that everyone has a kink, or has one they want eliminated, but an entire book could be written on this, and some kinks violate and exploit others). For the areas that remain open to change, this creative advantage, unique to humans, gifts a plasticity that departs from other great apes, chimpanzees being our closest genetic match.

We can embrace that life is organized energy, and, as humans, we have incredible influence over our emotional experience and energy, through our creative mind and imagination. The closer we can identify and match the truths of reality about how things work, the better our results. Our consciousness has been said to be a process of the universe perceiving itself. We can observe, create theories, and test what works in psychology and human relationships. The next step is to promote and share the winning formulas. We have discovered we have some access to our parasympathetic nervous system and endorphins. In qualifying the approach suggested in this book, it is a study in not getting stuck in pain. The message is a deliverance from an orientation toward unhappiness and poor self-esteem. We, as a species, are the most plastic.

28. FORMULA FOR MISTAKES

Homer gave me a formula for mistakes that I will share (not to make them... to deal with them).

Being human, I am going to fuck up. The best I can do is all I can do. People love to beat themselves up, always criticizing themselves. If we don't measure up to standards, the more we whip ourselves. Homer said people are afraid of not having guilt.

When people feel better, they do better. **When you make a mistake, you quickly acknowledge the mistake and say to yourself in a soothing voice, "I made a mistake and it is perfectly ok. Next time I will do better."** Immediately you will feel better and perform better. There is no value in beating oneself up, which will only increase the chances of more undesirable behaviour that flows from the bad feelings. **Feelings, thinking and behaviors improve when we are good to ourselves.** Obviously, this is not a license for deliberately doing wrong, but mistakes are a part of the human condition, and we need a strategy to deal with them. If an apology or restitution is needed, we can follow through with those.

It is stupid to call yourself stupid because of a mistake, because when you whine, your performance gets worse. Remind yourself that you're human and entitled to make a mistake. Past mistakes don't need to control our future but acknowledging them is necessary versus suppressing them. In this way they can be assimilated into your sense of self in a healthy manner. Failure to do so may compromise you in other ways since there is no escaping what your mind knows.

The most recent application I can think of for a minor mistake was from a member of the mastermind community I belong to. He was lamenting that he bombed a podcast. I asked him to consider the impossible situation of how a comedian could ever get back in the inspired place to entertain if they were down on themselves for misses. The freedom to make mistakes allows for expansion and increased creativity.

29. Stopping Self-Criticism

"Beware of perfection hissing 'not good enough' ... excellence is the opposite of perfection. It is the confidence to do the very best with what you currently have."
—*Joe Poni*

Anybody's problem is self-criticism and fear of self-criticism. It is *normal* but not healthy for people to be criticizing themselves all the time. "Well you did ok, but that could have been better." Harsh self-criticism causes anxiety and depression. "Everyone else is doing it so I don't know it is a mistake." Homer explained the following and said self-pity that results from self-criticism will ruin any plate of food. So how do we stop adding poison to our food?

The problem of putting ourselves down is universal. *Society* encourages it and the media encourages it. With everybody saying if you're not perfect you have a good reason to whine, how could you see it as a mistake? Just when I start to think I am just fine, I have a normal consciousness that says that is not the truth. "I'm not ok, there is something wrong with me." This is the sales pitch. He told me anything to make myself feel lousy I would buy. My history of criticizing myself was a familiar friend. The system (mirror) is working perfectly. It is working according to what I am telling myself. If I give my nervous system whining and crying orders it will respond.

Self-criticism is not a good thing. *Poor me* comes from self-criticism. Conventional wisdom says that guilt coming from self-criticism is a good voice that gets you back on track. Here we are arguing for the hammer again because we believe it has ribbons all over it. I can tell you this is not the truth. The more guilt I had about my eating disorder, the more I binged and purged. When we criticize ourselves, we rush to engage in more addictive behaviour. The cycle is self-perpetuating.

During periods when I was overweight, I was highly critical of myself. I thought I must lose weight, must be physically attractive, and it would be awful if I was unsuccessful, whining and screaming in my head. I thought that hating my fat body was an essential ingredient for having a trim body. I thought I was smart to feel guilty about it, and I also looked to those bad feelings to motivate me to diet. I was proud of my ability to disapprove of myself but crying from the pain at the same time. I was a person saying I wanted to feel good but arguing for feeling bad. If a person says, "I hate being overweight," they'll feel overweight and maybe be overweight. "I hate something" causes it. Homer said Dr. Albert Ellis would say it is not an eating problem but rather a thinking problem. The thought "I must watch my weight" carries the word *must*, which is the basis of all neurotic behaviour. He termed this musterbation. Thinking this way gives a person stress and makes them want to eat. Hating the fat body is what keeps the body fat. Homer says while we are busy feeling guilt that we should do better, behaviour and feelings get worse. Increasing pain is not an effective approach to getting over addiction.

The way out is to love my overweight body. I resisted loving my overweight body because in my mind I had an ego based on hating it. (Remember, all feelings and behavior are generated by our belief about what is smart or stupid.) You can't walk through a door with the sign "stupid" even though it could lead to happiness. In my mind, I thought it was stupid to love my fat body, therefore I was resisting it even though it was the solution to my happiness. It was my hating my overweight body that caused me to be overweight. He encouraged me to love my overweight body just the way it was. Thinking after I get trim I will be happy doesn't work. I have to be happy now. Loving what is, my fat body, is the only way out of unhappiness. Loving *what is* gets happiness now. "I am perfectly fine the way I am. I am womanly and feminine." "I'm proud of being overweight" goes against the old religion of hating. I could say, "I prefer to be slender, but I don't need to be slender, and it's not awful if I'm not." It was my mind that caused me to overeat, not my body. It is a superstitious belief that hating will prevent it. We wished that hating worked, but it is no more than wishful thinking. Fear, hate, and shame will die if I love my overweight body.

Shame and hate are buddies. I'm proud of them but complaining about them. They will die if I love my body. Loving my fat body is smart because it relaxes me and my body responds by becoming thin. When you love with all your heart, there is no hate or unhappiness, which drives emotional eating. Homer reminded me that anybody's body is beautiful. The problem is never the body. The mistake is criticizing and whining. "Well I did ok, but I could have done better," always postponing happiness. Thought always comes before the feeling. He warned me the whining wants to argue and will argue for itself. He said there was no rational argument, the body is beautiful the way it is.

It annoys me that some people feel the need to comment on weight. (Body shaming) It is so easy to point the finger and assume that someone who has a high BMI is unhappy. Whether such a person is struggling or self-accepting, it is assumed they are struggling and are targets for ridicule. Ridicule has never helped anyone, and many people struggle in less visible ways. People who have a high BMI and struggle with the psychology behind it must think to themselves, "What about all the people who have neurotic issues and effectively hide it from the scrutiny of others?"

He also tackled the issue through the happiness anxiety paradigm. He chastised me saying, "Don't let me get rid of my problems," recognizing that part of my mind wanted to be unhappy. I was not used to not having a problem. Echoing Byron Katie's book title *Who Would You be Without Your Story*, he asked, "Who would you be without your problems?" and then followed it up by saying, "I would be a beautiful woman full of self-confidence for any situation."

If you really hate something you don't do it. If you sincerely want a slender body, you do not overeat. "I'm going to do this if it kills me," not literally, but emphasis and conviction wise. Homer said that I loved my friend shame, and fat was my ticket to shame. Therefore, the desire to overeat is a subconscious desire to feel shame and humiliation. The sick mind lies and gets away with it. I must eat because "I love it so much" is a lie. The evidence was that I wanted to feel shame, my familiar old friend. (Interestingly humiliation and shame were predominant emotions for me as a young teenager when I felt my breasts were too large.) I want fat not because I like fat, but it's my excuse for shame. I thought that if I lost shame something bad would happen. I praise my guilt and shame—that's my religion. I went to church every day to worship my shame.

This concept is very powerful. **"If a person keeps going down the road and getting the same result, the reason for going down the road is the result."** This is a statement from Homer that has great implications for the addiction world, and it has stayed in the front of my mind.

TWO DOORS OUT OF SHAME

1.   Don't overeat.

2.   Say that being overweight is not terrible.

Refusing both doors is proof I am having a love affair with shame.

Additional insight and leverage comes from the awareness that we are making a sales pitch in our head when we are walking by the fridge. We are saying that food is *comforting*. We never have only an event but are dealing with an irrational or rational sales pitch. This is true of many addictions. You played the innocent victim while you told the sales lady to say cake is a great comfort or diversion. I feel bored or frustrated so the cake is going to comfort me. The cake is getting away with lying! Getting more food will get happiness is a lie. If I learn to think happy now, I don't reach for food to get happy. It is my own thinking that relaxes me as I approve of myself before eating, affirming eating cake will relax me. I could sit down and close my eyes and get good feelings without the negative effects. This is a nice escape without any bad things. I like being quiet and still and I am being nice to myself and feel smart by doing it this way. It's healthy to want to be away from feelings of pressure. With cake, I am saying "stupid," and my mind is divided. Before we do the addictive *thing*, there is generally the internal dialogue that says, "This is smart and this is dumb."

Again... If a person keeps going down a road and getting the same result, the reason for going down the road is the result. Can you relate to this idea?. Addictions almost always have a negative side effect. Let's take for example the gambler who chases the high of winning. At first glance, it would appear this is solely driving the addiction. The gambler's life falling apart is not seen, by most, as anything other than a bad consequence. Quite possibly the bad consequences are satisfying a secondary addiction to shame. This is why I wanted to have your attention on the issue of happiness anxiety at the start of Part Two. If you have an unwritten script that dictates happiness is not right for you, you are beat before you start. There will be an invisible ceiling on your happiness/success.

Homer says ambivalence alone can lead toward overeating and other addictive behaviours. This conflict over loving/hating bingeing is the ambivalence. "I love this bingeing, but I hate it." If I only love it or hate it, I will not do it. Homer makes an important distinction between the whining kind of hating versus the hating with a tone of anger. Sometimes we say "I hate" with a barking tone. It is a different kind of anger, not "I hate" with a whine. The whining kind of anger is passive and dependent. The hate with a barking tone is not passive and is action driven. So if I genuinely hate something, I don't do it. If I love it and hate it, it increases tension, and one addiction will be replaced for another. Traditionally, people have thought the way to get over addiction is to increase pain. He states that having affection for something is the way to get over addiction. "Thank you for the years of comfort." Gratitude.

If I am totally positive about cake, I eat it slowly and enjoy it.
If I am completely negative about cake, I don't eat it.

He said the more pleasure I get from eating the less I will eat, and the weight takes care of itself. This is helped by slowing down. The "hurry up" was anxiety, not pleasure. Less is better, more is not better. I love eating cake enables more enjoyment and eating less because of enjoyment.

Bingeing and Purging

Homer brought up again that two words explain all human behavior and emotion—smart and stupid. In order to binge and purge, I had to believe it was smart or I could not do it. He said when you see bingeing as stupid, you will lose the desire. Desire comes from the attitude that it is smart. **If you kill the desire, you don't need willpower at all.**

He used the example of drinking alcohol. A person thinks, "When I drink I feel better right away and that is smart." So the immediate comfort is smart. Also the drinker says, "Well I realize it would be a stronger thing for me to turn down alcohol, but I am a weak person." "It's smart for me to be the weak person that I am when thinking drinking alcohol is smart."

The same goes for smoking. That's why the smoker gets comfort. He or she says it is a smart and calming thing, believing the propaganda, born gullible. The smoker is approving of themselves. There is nothing flawed about seeking comfort or desire to escape from pressure; however, the methods we choose are important. There is nothing calming about smoking. It's the thinking that gives a degree of comfort. Many people have been killed by smoking. When he or she smokes, the smoker gets a temporary lift. Smoking gets the credit, but smoking doesn't do one nice thing. Three weeks after quitting smoking, the ex-smoker still believes the brainwashing that the smoker has something nice. It is tempting to rationalize and defend things that provide a temporary escape, but we cannot ever escape the consequences of our choices.

You approve of yourself for doing the things you label as comforting right before you engage. We engage and think it is "smart under these conditions." We feel stressed or deprived because of criticizing ourselves in other areas, so addictive behavior comforts us and compensates us. We need to find out what we are criticizing ourselves about, become aware of what we are telling ourselves, and praise ourselves instead. We want to get some leverage over our thoughts before we start reaching for the fix. If I didn't have guilt and fear, I wouldn't be bingeing and purging.

If we don't intervene before reaching for the fix, we praise ourselves just before engaging, but we don't continue with praise, or at least not whole heartedly. The other voice says this is a sign of failure. The thought that excessive or inappropriate eating is going to comfort me is not true and there is some degree of resistance/guilt. So again, the ambiguity of loving and hating is present. I was saying I hated the bingeing and purging, but that was not the whole story. I also loved it but was not fully admitting that. Telling myself I hated it was merely whining because genuine hating would make me stop.

I would not have a problem if I didn't feel guilty about bingeing and purging. If I really praised myself and said, "I love bingeing and purging," I would lose the desire to binge and purge because of the constant and consistent praising of myself and therefore feeling happy.

I have been saying, "I hate that I put my health at risk by purging. I want my kids to have a mother." (whining and hating)

Homer instructed me to tell myself I love purging, which will weaken my desire to do it. He said hating in this case is whining. I was feeling unfamiliar with unconditional love, weak in loving but good at hating. He said he wanted me to binge and purge when I think about it and instantly add the thought, "I love to binge and purge," to be proud of my ability to do exactly as I want. Having affection for something is the way to get over addiction. Whining hate causes the dependency. When you enjoy something, you can let go. When you don't enjoy something, you get hung up.

30. Treating Inferiority

I am going to talk about how I was helped to make peace with being inferior. I had great difficulty in school and always felt like learning was beyond me. The personal experience of feeling inferior was magnified one hundred times after my psychosis resolved. As I mentioned, I felt subhuman. It was during this time when I was so consumed with feelings of being less than every person alive that I finally faced I had a learning disability as well.

I also recognized that I had poor organizational skills and poor short-term memory. I recalled my summers working as a waitress where other waitresses could easily manage six tables and four tables was my limit. This experience was more proof for me. There was no other option than facing my inferiority. With this inferiority came deep shame of myself. I was in complete overwhelm.

Homer addressed my predominant thought, which was "I am inferior to everybody and I hate it." He said I believed the thought was the problem, but it was my hating the thought that was the problem.

The first thing I learned from him was that no amount of hate or shame was going to magically take my inadequacies away. I had attached virtue to my hate habit. I felt proud of my ability to hate being inferior. He also told me I loved my friend *shame*. I was having a love affair with shame. He said shame is not a friend. It is shit masquerading as a virtue. Shame how we talk, how we don't talk, how we look, how we perform. "Look everyone, I'm ashamed of myself." Being inferior is not the problem, it is the shame I attached.

We had a discussion about weakness when exploring this. He said there is no shame in weakness...not a drop, until we put it there. He qualified that sometimes it is desirable to be strong, but there is no shame in weakness itself.

Homer said he was going to teach me a new way to think. This new way of thinking was like a new dress. Everything I had worn up until then had not felt comfortable. The new dress was comfortable but a bit unfamiliar at first so I would want to take it off saying "this is not me." Heaven seemed strange and a degree uncomfortable. I was trapped in jail with my thinking. He said we need to outsmart the part of the mind that wants to be unhappy. He explained my pain always comes from my whining tone of voice. Usually the desire to whine is more clever. He said the magician is very good at getting the audience to look away while it puts the rabbit in the hat. I use circumstances as excuses for whining, and I whine because I want to, out of habit. All my life, I have been whining because I thought whining was a smart thing to do. Everyone else is whining, and I would be stupid if I did not whine under these circumstances. We've all been brainwashed that we should whine.

The statement:

"I am inferior."
The sales pitch: "I hate that I am inferior." "I shouldn't be inferior in everything I do, friend, mother." (whining, crying, screaming)
Changed sales pitch: "I love it that I am inferior, it is perfectly ok to be inferior, glad I am different." "Yes I am inferior, and it gives me depth." "I love it that everyone is better than me."
"I am inferior, no reason I should be perfect."
"I am willing to be inferior... (creates openness, no stress or frustration)."

No whining about it. Never say "I'm inferior" again in a whining tone.

The old habit doesn't want me to do that. The mind will fight for what is familiar. He said, "Don't whine and say, 'I can't stand being inferior,' but rather 'I am so glad I am inferior.'" What has given me the pain is "I shouldn't be," "It's awful to be," and "I can't stand," all whining. "I'm so glad" erases "hating."

He said I am the boss of my tone of voice in my head and I needed to practice it with energy and pleasure. If we start to complain, the boss (our new insight) is going to say, "Stop it." We are not going to be just interested in *poor me*. We can even practice dealing with self-pity. Self-pity keeps showing up at the door because we keep letting it in. We can put self-pity at the door on purpose and slam the door in its face. He said this would become more automatic with practice.

People are unfamiliar with unconditional love. We are weak in loving but good at hating. People believe hating has power somehow. You are not loving yourself when you are whining, and you are creating pain. When we come up short, our tendency is to argue for the hammer, which is hate and complaining. We think it is *smart* to complain. These are the ribbons we put all over the hammer. If we are not perfect, we are calling ourselves a failure because of perfectionist standards. He said we go after pain because it is a habit, and we get some degree of comfort by patting ourselves on the head about being virtuous. Lastly, we don't clearly see a better way.

He explained to me that when there is no whining, we deal with the situation quite well. By that he meant, "I may have the practical problems of dealing with having a mental illness and lower intelligence, but no emotional problem. Big deal if I need more time to learn a task or require help." This is how to be in a harmonious relationship with oneself. I will use the brain I have, at full capacity.

There is a favourite online animator/comedian of Calvin's who we often listen to. His name is Zach Hadel. His username is Psychicpebbles. His podcasts include Sleeypcast and Schmucks. He began in 2009 on Newgrounds. He presently has 1.9 million subscribers on YouTube. Zach has some degree of a speech impediment. He sounds as though he is talking through his nose. He does not care, and he is amazing. He operates from a high level of self-esteem and passion. Zach actually uses his voice to his advantage to speak in different character voices for improvisational comedy. He does an excellent Donald Trump. Nothing breaks his stride, and he has zero shame.

31. Unstoppable Self-Esteem

"Never be afraid to shine. Remember the sun doesn't give a fuck if it blinds you."
—*Author Unknown*

I am going to teach you how to praise yourself as I learned from Homer. Homer teaches the secret of happiness is approving of the self regardless of performance. We are told pride is a bad thing and not to be so "stuck on yourself." Self-praise and bragging on yourself are good things. We want to pat ourselves on the back. Homer explicitly said you can't praise yourself too much.

If you are solid in your pride, others will change very quickly. Others may initially test and bristle at you feeling you are Mrs. or Mr. Perfect. You convey that if they adjust to that, there won't be any problems. You are who you are with no apologies.

Pride is the solution to all problems because it gets you out of pain, and you perform better when you feel better. Praise is in the self. There is nothing you can say against pride. Focus on the qualities and virtues you already have. Nobody was made good by being told they are bad.

Homer explained praising yourself is like a brand new blouse. It is unfamiliar at first, so you want to take it off. Put the urge aside temporarily. You don't have to think of it as a permanent thing, you can alway take off the blouse and go back to hell. Healthy self-esteem for me comes from valuing highly what I do have and keeps me very happy. I am changing my religion. I am proud of me, my body, my mental illness history, and my intellect. He said your new friend "pride" replaces your old friend "shame." You cannot be too proud. If you go straight to positives and focus on the positives, it takes care of the awfulizing. When you do positive thinking, it all looks good. Circumstances don't have anything to do with it.

Homer uses the metaphor of wearing a small crown instead of a large glistening one. The large glistening crown looks so great, but it is so heavy. It requires other people to hold it up. A smaller crown is so light we can hold it up with our own self-talk and approval. So having a small crown gives you a weak dependence on other people so that you don't care whether they like you or not. The irony is the more you like yourself the more others want to help you hold up your crown (McDonald, 1999-2006).

It's really nobody's business what you think of yourself. Flex on yourself!

32. A Movement

"The friction between what is vs. what can be is the burn that drives change."
—Michael Rowell

The following is a repurposing of Homer's work with me, but a worthy cause, and gives the book two goals. I can imagine his confident laugh cheering me on.

Where shame used to originate behind the walls of asylums it now originates from pages inside the DSM and its progeny. The DSM-5 which is as clinically cold as an asylum and equally unapologetic feels like the final confirmation of a life sentence of suffering, medications and shame. I doubt it has a disclaimer for the shame it invokes. Nobody in their right mind would take it on as a final boss and most resign to a life of shame. The DSM is deeply established, supported and referenced in the psych community and the cornerstone of the medical model. It has been challenged on grounds of its power to cause shame if it extends its reach and captures more deviance, unnecessarily. The DSM needs to be careful not to become too ambitious, to prevent its own undoing. If everyone is represented by disorder it cannot shame anyone. The only other way to win with the DSM is to make shame disappear.

Biologically, shame is merely another tool to support life, fashioned by evolution. It has survival value for social cohesion. We can even observe it in great apes and dogs. It functions to regulate behavior for survival where there is a need for cooperation. In humans it presents in a couple ways. Social anxiety sweat signals others because it is malodorous. I don't think this is a mistake. You can compare it to thermoregulation sweat which is non pugnacious. Therefore, it is easy to conclude evolution selected it for a function. It is submissive and communicates the individual is not in an alpha position. Today, we, as a species, are more independent compared to our early ancestors so shame has less value for our survival. It is good to tell shame to 'sit down' where survival is tested less. What is natural to humans is designing and implementing change, which may include saying 'no' to some of our tendencies. (I will spare the social blush since it seems to have a sexual function).

YOUR BRAND NEW SHIRT

With an attitude of embracing and celebrating both our strengths and weaknesses, we can reject shame and mental illness stigma. Shame cripples and distracts us from discovering what needs healing. Your new friend "pride" is replacing your old friend "shame". Let's build momentum. It is important for every person with a mental illness history to be in this position. Collectively, if people can reject mental illness shame, it loses stigma one person at a time. We have come a long way from the term "insane" and its negative connotations. I personally believe many people, professionals, clinics, and hospitals favour the verbiage "mental health" vs. "mental illness" because of stigma pressure. Using the word "mental health" when we mean "mental illness" is like shy flirting. We can speak directly. Mental health and mental illness are complete opposites. The emerging trend is toward acceptance vs. tolerance and exclusion. We can cancel mental illness shame. We can empower ourselves and those we love! Shame derives power from ignorance and fear and has been the status quo for far too long. We can do more than push back. *I want you to take the leap and celebrate mental illness, non sheepishly, non defensively, but boldly...like you won a medal! No shy flirting!* Taking it to social media with the word *illness* proves healing, strength and acceptance, bar none.

#CELEBRATEMENTALILLNESS

Here is a question from a member of the mastermind community I belong to who agreed with de-stigmatizing mental illness:

How can we celebrate mental illness? Isn't the goal to resolve mental illness so we can enjoy the freedom that a healthy mind affords?

I can appreciate the confusion and need for clarification. It is precisely celebrating my psychosis history that moved me from the most crippling depression of my life into happiness and high self-esteem. This was in sharp contrast to my self-criticism, guilt, shame, and whining habits. Accepting, praising, and celebrating myself for my human weaknesses is the opposite of pressuring myself and demanding reality be different or saying that it "shouldn't be". The "goal" is acceptance about whatever is going on without adding shame, in particular. People attach virtue to habits like self-criticism, worry, shame, guilt, and whining. For example, 'It would be stupid not to whine under the conditions of mental illness'. So people are defending these habits but crying from the pain. Thinking, feelings, and behavior improve when we praise ourselves. This has protective and healing features. I weigh the nurture side of the nurture/nature paradigm quite heavily in the development of mental illness. I acknowledge a genetic predisposition, in some cases. I was treated under the medical model and took psychotropic medication for psychosis while in hospital, and for some years afterward. Antidepressants were contraindicated for me, so I was forced to find answers outside the medical model to heal paralyzing depression and a self-esteem left in shreds. The question I faced was how can I experience high self-esteem and happiness with a severe mental illness history? The answer was both the help and the cure.

33. Everyday Applications

"Is it just me, or am I really getting weirder and hotter as time goes by?"
—Secret Smiles Personal Blog

I apply Homer's techniques to "treat" my negative feelings when they occur. I am not going to lie, I often have some anxiety when I am meeting a new client. Keep in mind, I have already screened my clients, stay out of sketchy areas, and often go to new appointments with a drive from my bodyguard boyfriend. I say to myself in a soothing voice, "I am anxious right now, and that is perfectly ok. I am human, and my fears will gradually go away."

Here is a list of other non-whining statements:

"I want people to criticize me if they want to."
"I look forward to my boyfriend's moods."
"I am glad I am inferior to others; they can do the jobs I don't want to do."
"I am so glad I am not a tolerant person, that is my confidence showing."
"I am so glad my neighbour spits repetitively every time he sees me outside, it is amusing." (true story)
"I am proud of my aging body."
"It is great that other women are prettier."
"I celebrate my mate leaving me; he should do what he wants with his life."

"I am glad they see I am shy."

"I want my child to be a dreamer because he likes it."

"I am willing to have another psychotic break."

"Yes I am an imperfect mother, I fucked up, so what?"

"I can stutter and it is perfectly ok."

"It's fun to be upset."

"I've been to hell and back. Coming back was a big achievement."

"I am willing to feel dissociated."

"Breakup? I can do that."

"I slipped back to overeating, excellent, excellent."

"I embarrassed myself today. It is perfectly ok. Tomorrow I will do better."

(If I lose my license, I will buy a dirtbike and get a helmet with earphones)

Since I mentioned I was allowed emotions in measured amounts while growing up, I sometimes come up against my own happiness anxiety. I am absolutely at my happiest joking around with my children, and we are downright silly by spells. As I approach high levels of happiness, I sometimes start taking my mental health temperature with the thought, "What if I am so happy I become manic and psychotic again?" A complete buzzkill. First, I might mention that my psychiatrist reassured me that when you are off your rocker you generally don't ask yourself if you are off your rocker (my words). Secondly, I remind myself that I had some negative programming around happiness and that it is not the end of the world if I do become psychotic again. I have a right to be happy, and it is very good for my children. This removes the invisible ceiling on my happiness.

The formula is to start where you are without any pressure for things to be different and have a soothing tone of voice in your head. Calvin was obsessing about his physical features, and I mentioned to him that Grandma said, "If you have a round face you need to make it square and vice versa", never satisfied. I told him to stop adding pain to his artistic perfectionism. He is, by nature, detail-oriented. There is nothing *bad* about being a perfectionist. I encouraged him to *start* there. "I am neurotically concerned about my appearance and that is ok". Then maybe he can have a look later on at "needing" to have reality a certain way. He, like all of us, is just a peon here on earth, and reality is not going to bend for us. He is doubling his pain by adding that he 'shouldn't be a perfectionist' about his looks. If he *plays* with this a bit, he will find that he has tremendous power and control to employ his perfectionism where he wants and mute it in other places. I personally like being a perfectionist, knowing exactly what I like and being super clear about it. It has some downfalls, but it certainly has its good points, too. The ability to play without being too attached to the outcome, is where the power lies.

For anxiety in general, the technique of saying things positively in one's head lowers anxiety faster. Anybody with a history of an anxiety disorder will recognize anxiety can appear and it is doubled by thinking "it is terrible to be experiencing it." It is a case of feeling bad because you feel bad. I want you to *start where you are.* "I'm glad I'm nervous." This formula interrupts that escalation, and my experience is that my anxiety is acceptable. It eliminated the frequency of my stuttering as well. One powerful approach, which works well for me, is saying things like, "Sweaty hands, yes I can do that!" "Feeling shaky, yes I can do that!" "Anxiety, yes I can do that!"

I want you to be patient and gentle with yourself while you are still learning about not *needing* reality to be a certain way. As you start to realize that things are a *preference* rather than a *need*, you will be happier and roll with things better. Admittedly, this is a learning curve. I want you to understand at times you may need to simply say to yourself in a soothing voice, "Right now I am feeling terrible and that is perfectly ok, I am human." (Alternatively you can focus on a soothing emotion like affection in response to something negative. You cannot feel stressed while concentrating on the word "affection." It is very effective and I have used it.) This may be the case as you are learning and also at times when you are faced with multiple or major issues. After a spell of this gentle acceptance, you can remind yourself that you don't *need* reality to be a certain way. It will work. Sometimes you can go back and forth between the gentle statement and then challenging your beliefs about needing things to be a certain way.

There will be situations where you may need to act on a reality that is beyond your ability to live with. An example that comes to mind could be someone you live with who has a drug addiction. For your well being, you may need to have the person move out. You are still free to treat your feelings about that reality, however, and I would encourage you to.

Everyday Applications

We all experience setbacks. If and when I experience setbacks with smoking or bulimia, I am going to reconquer them in the following way. I know you already know the answer to this... consistent and constant praise of myself. I will praise myself for doing what I want to do. By avoiding the self-criticism and guilt rabbit hole and praising myself instead, calling myself a success for doing what I want to do, I will be able to feel better quickly and be on the path to better straight away.

I have some valuable Bob Proctor ideas I keep fresh in my mind. Bob has said that it is useful to write problems on a piece of paper so the problem is not in you anymore. It would seem this keeps it objective. Also, Bob talked about Napoleon Hill's task of looking in the mirror when affirming goals. You can't hide from yourself in the mirror, and there are no distractions. It is a place of honesty (Proctor, 2015).

I would like to mention victimhood. Since my teenage years, there has been a trend toward victim culture. Many people over identify with being a victim and it subverts their happiness and keeps them stuck. I do not intend to minimize people's experience of suffering. I understand mental illness. What I hope is that you can move away from feeling like a victim. When people strongly identify with being a victim, it cripples their ability to see actions possible to make their life better. We don't want to kick the can further down the street. Staying a victim is passive and dangerous to one's well being. Nathaniel Branden told me that a person would not act helpless on a deserted island.

As I mentioned, Amber is going through some gender identity issues. She experiences negativity in school from this. I encourage her to share and resist becoming a victim and to forge her internal confidence. We talk a lot and infuse humour where appropriate. Calvin showed us a hilarious video called "Gay Frogs with Alex Jones." The video mocks Alex Jones reacting negatively to being gay. Amber is going to crush the art world and uses art as therapy and a passion outlet.

34. LOVE AND HAPPINESS

"Self-love comes before neighbour love."
—Homer McDonald

I would not feel I finished this book unless I captured some of the things Homer said on the issue of romantic love. His two books *Stop Your Divorce* and *Advanced Sessions* are the best books I have ever read. I just wanted to mention highlights from those books that will support your happiness.

In his book *Stop Your Divorce*, Homer said the important thing to understand about love is that it is centered around pride (McDonald, 1999-2006). We carry our own level of self-esteem and pride into our relationships and are most compatible with partners who share a similar level of self-esteem. Homer explained people aren't attracted to others they are "ashamed of" (McDonald, 1999-2006, p. 22). In support of this, he stated that we need to be individuals who are concerned about nurturing our own pride and our partner's pride. "Happy people who are in love are a mutual admiration society" (McDonald, 1999-2006, p. 21).

"Criticizing, complaining, arguing, and showing jealousy are the worst things we can do, because that is experienced as an attack on both people's pride" (McDonald, 1999-2006, p. 22). All these behaviors kill attraction and undermine pride because they make us needy. The more needy we are, the less our mate respects us. If you experience intense emotions like the impulse to cling, or display moodiness, or any other pressuring behavior, give yourself some space away from your partner so you can collect yourself. In this space, you can think about what affect your behavior will have on your partner in terms of pride. It will help you gain composure and not act out on your emotions. The obvious result will be an increase in your own dignity and your partner's pride in you (McDonald, 1999-2006).

McDonald (1999-2006) and Dale Carnegie talked about not criticizing people. "Criticism is dangerous because it wounds a person's precious pride, hurts his sense of importance, and arouses resentment" (Carnegie, 1981, p. 5). Carnegie says it is a hollow victory, at best, when we "appear" to argue and win. Homer warned how any time we attack a partner's beliefs, friends, choice of music, etc., it is damaging because our partner's pride is tied up in those things (McDonald, 1999-2006). Criticizing can be tempting, but it is contrary to your goals for closeness. I saw a funny meme once that said, "My husband and I play this fun game called *why do you do it that way?* And there are no winners."

Homer said, criticizing is damaging to a relationship (McDonald, 1999-2006). You can think in business terms. One bad review has to be buried under at least ten good reviews. Carnegie says, "The little word 'my' is the most important one in human affairs, and properly to reckon with it is the beginning of wisdom. It has the same force whether it is 'my dinner,' 'my dog,' 'my house,' or 'my father'" (Carnegie, 1981, p. 127). To illustrate, I know everyone can identify with the idea that we can say something critical about our family, but if anyone else does... look out. We find it highly offensive. If you don't want to invite distance into your relationship, don't criticize.

Homer wrote, "Give your partner complete freedom. The way to get him over ice cream is to give him all the ice cream he wants" (McDonald, 2010, p. 89). You don't have to fear that you are going to lose your partner with this mindset because you are believing in yourself. Your security is your most attractive trait. If your partner is flirting, it is fine. Homer told me when you pressure and chase your mate, they inevitably move away from you. He said crying and fighting are not going to build a happy relationship. "Does it build a wife's pride to be with a husband who complains, who says over and over I'm a baby? Does this turn her on? No" (McDonald, 1999-2006, p. 57).

Homer explains in both his books *Stop Your Divorce* and *Advanced Sessions* that the greatest asset we can bring to our romantic lives is understanding that we don't actually need love. He said, "The more we believe we need it the less we are going to have it" (McDonald, 1999-2006, p. 17). People don't want the pressure from a partner who "needs." When we focus on what we would like instead of exaggerating it to a need, we are easy to be with. We naturally take on a secure vibe, which is sexy.

A final discussion from Homer on nurturing our relationships is to keep our interests outside the relationship. This makes us fulfilled and interesting and builds our pride and, therefore, our partner's pride in us (McDonald,1999-2006). My mom had a busy social life and was involved in volunteer activities. She was interesting to my dad. Remember I said I would mention one of the ways my dad's lack of worrying helped him? It was this attitude of being laid back that attracted my mom to him in the first place. She was eighteen years younger and very beautiful. She told me she asked my dad, "Don't you worry about where I am when I am gone?" His reply was, "As long as you know where you are." My dad embodied the concept of giving total freedom, and my mom never left him. They loved each other, and my mom spent hours with my dad at the nursing home every day before he passed.

I mentioned earlier that my personal pattern was to leave relationships after I felt my partner was conquered and no longer a challenge. By studying Homer, I understand that this was a form of poor self-esteem where I looked down on anybody for being in love with me because I thought so little of myself. It happened at a subconscious level whereby my subconscious wanted a challenge in order to feel passion (McDonald, 1999-2006). As my self-esteem has improved, I can accept love. (If you happen to be on the reverse end of this, the simplified answer is to stay a bit outside of your partner's reach.)

When I first contacted Homer back in 2007, it was after I had found his book *Stop Your Divorce.* I am going to share some personal things he said to me on the issue of romance over the years. These discussions were around James and myself.

After the psychosis had resolved, there was a period before I moved back into the family home. Homer counselled me to just agree if James brought up serious talk. He said to listen and show respect, understanding, and thanks for sharing whatever it is. He said you can bring up serious talk if you know how to handle it. (In his book *Stop Your Divorce*, he cautioned against serious talk because oftentimes serious talk develops into criticism and pressure.) He said to act happy all the time and date other men. He said no woman ever gets her husband back unless she's dating another man is what research shows. A disloyal one always gets the husband back if she doesn't drop her boyfriend too fast. The husband needs competition. People are often defensive about anything perceived as "game playing," but I am going to quote Homer to answer this. "People say, 'Be true to yourself,' I say, 'Which self? The self that wants to shoot at the ground and end in self-pity or the self that wants to hit the bull's-eye and win my goal?'" (McDonald, 1999-2006, p. 67). We always have choices about how we conduct ourselves around others, and if we are honest, it is not always in our best interest to allow feelings to dictate our behavior.

He said when you have a new relationship, hold back on the quantity but not the quality. The space between is important, going over things in one's imagination. Familiarity breeds contempt. Upping quantity decreases quality. You don't have to tone down the excitement. He said putting focus on quantity, eating more, fast, and wanting more is the opposite of relaxing and enjoying more. The focus should not be on "give me more." Many people ruin their marriages with the attitude "give me more." They say, "I am content, but I don't have passion"... the part of the mind that wants discontent. He said marriage in order to be good does not need to be exciting. The wife who makes her husband her only source of pleasure drives him nuts because she is insecure. More is not better, less is better.

During those days before James took me back, Homer talked to me about holding back on sex based on my psychiatrist's recommendation that it was not just fun and games for me. Homer said that James had wanted sex without earning it and it "was my duty" in his mind. "I'm a failure as a man if I don't get it, and she's a bad woman if she's not giving it." Homer said after James gives me attention I can give him praise. He said praise is more important than sex. He said two people can have sex and one rolls over and says, "That duty is done." We don't want sex as much as the praise.

He said people can be happily married if they decide to never complain. Most people are trying to steal; thieves trying to run the other person's life. He says protect the other person's ego, never complain and be lavish in praise. Most people like to point out where their mate is wrong. "Look how smart I am. I can see my mate did this wrong. I can see what is better." Don't complain about anything, ever. If I praise him and tell him he's stupid, there's too much sand in the ice cream for him to enjoy the ice cream.

Once I had moved back, there were a few other bumpy patches.

Homer counselled me on (1) being taken for granted by James, and (2) his moodiness. He said I could put a positive slant on the situation. Resistance gives me pain, so my willingness to be taken for granted was the solution. He said people want what they can't have and don't want what they can have. People have low self-esteem, and they look down on what they own (furniture, wife, car). "I want him to see me as reliable. I'm glad that he is taking me for granted." "I'm glad for him to be doing whatever he is doing." This empowers me, and now I will do something new and different. This is a non-passive approach to feeling good and places the responsibility for that within one's own control.

He said the perfect solution was to enjoy my freedom, enjoy other men and their attention. The unconquered person gets more than the conquered, more catering. He also reminded me that I was not "deprived of attention." He said this would build my confidence and happiness and motivate James to give me what I wanted. **The assumption is that while acceptance is a good thing, we assume it means no action or continuing to endure.** Rather, "I am so glad about reality, and I know how to get attention from others. This way I am not pressuring my mate." People never get what they strongly desire (not being taken for granted)—desiring it works against getting it. Complaining about the present situation disqualifies me from better situations.

He said my feelings in my stomach about his moodiness came from what I told myself in my head. Here is what he proposed to outsmart self-pity. He said self-pity will call the solution stupid.

1. x is happening.
2. I don't want x.
3. Therefore I have a problem.
4. I want x equals no problem.

Saying I want x is going against society's command. It is a normal thing for me to not like it or not want it when he is moody. If I want him to be moody, I don't have a problem. The old me that loved to suffer minded that. Confronting someone about a bad mood is like saying, "You know I can't be happy unless you are happy." He also said James was punishing me because he knew it bothered me. When he sees it doesn't bother me, he will stop. He could hide his moodiness from me, but that would destroy his motivation. The reason I want him to be moody is because he is. It's his life. He should spend it the way he wants. He wants to be moody because he is getting self-righteous pleasure. Good for him; he is doing what he wants and now I'll do what I want to do. When you allow the other person's behavior to upset you, they get worse. Your complaining adds to the problem.

The other part was my concern that the moodiness was a symptom of general discontent and James was going to end the relationship and I still wanted to preserve the family. Homer said a conscious fear is often a subconscious wish. Homer said he was counselling a man who was afraid his wife would divorce him. Fear says, "I'm your friend, and I want to protect you." Fear makes him suspicious, critical, and a whiner, so he drives her away. He wants to drive her away—she's his excuse for being unhappy.

The belief that wanting something is going to get it is mistaken. Homer used the example of the husband saying his wife would not give him a chance to show he had changed. "If she will just give me what I want, I will prove I am not spoiled." The only way you can prove is by being happy while not getting your own way. For me, it was better to have an attitude of "I would be happy if James left me." When you say, "I'm afraid of x," you will get x. If I want a divorce, my mate won't divorce me. Men never leave a happy woman, a woman who wants him to leave, if she's happy about wanting him to leave. Act like you're a happy person whether you feel it or not. Not to keep him, but it moves you toward feeling happy, which is more important than keeping him. In my case, he said I could be happy with him or happy without him because the feeling in my stomach comes from what I tell myself in my head. When I tell myself it is stupid to whine, my stomach feels good. I am the only person who can hurt me or make myself feel good. (Homer's books are far superior to my jot notes streaming from his mind. I encourage you to read his work. The *Advanced Sessions* seem hard to find. I sold my Lexus hastily, and his prized CDs went with it. Every time I would listen to them, I would learn something different. He had a passionate and great speaking voice.)

Homer and Nathaniel had opposing views on 'mystery', as it relates to romantic love.

Nathaniel's position was, "How can there be love without sight", further arguing we do not love indiscriminately in romantic love so we need to identify the uniqueness in an individual. He said people naturally come with enough mystery without adding more. Homer's position was *less is more*. He said that because passion originates in the subconscious, staying just slightly in the unconquered position keeps the subconscious engaged. I personally want nothing to do with a dead mouse dropped at my doorstep. Homer and Nathaniel also differed on how to achieve self-esteem. Nathaniel deconstructed self-esteem so people could know how to behave to generate the experience. Homer believed we can have it straight away, and, therefore, we do better when we feel better. I say we naturally will satisfy Nathaniel's six pillars by this approach. As I mentioned before, Nathaniel's work in the *Disowned Self* is very valuable, and I think it is especially important for individuals who have a mental illness history. It opens the door to greater self-discovery, which can then be assimilated comfortably into one's self-concept. Insight is always good. I am chomping at the bit to share my contribution around insight in my next book.

35. ABUSE

A word on tolerating abuse. Abuse is never ok. It is not ok to tolerate it or abuse another person. Domestic abuse is an escalating, insidious, and dangerous situation. Never apply the ideas of "accepting" put forth in this book with regard to abuse. Beware and seek help if you are being abused or are abusing.

36. Status Update

"All these puzzles are only thinking problems, whether to do with socializing, can't control my eating, husband is going to leave me."
—Homer McDonald

Arguably Homer was pro getting rid of negative feelings as quickly as possible. He mentioned in his book *Stop Your Divorce* that he was criticized sometimes for advocating an "unfeeling" mindset. He addressed this in a couple of different ways. He said by using your head, you "will be a feeling person with happy feelings rather than depressed or hurt feelings" (McDonald, 1999-2006, p. 47). He also used a gardener metaphor where he said weeds were choking out the roses and that the proper procedure would be to remove the weeds that were using up resources. This action would not mean the gardener was against plants (McDonald, 1999-2006).

With Homer the teacher, and me the student, we outperformed the DSM-5. One of the things my dad said was, "Someday she is going to come up against a brick wall." Also my dad, "When you're coming out of a turn, step on the gas." I am 95% free of symptoms of dissociation. I rarely binge and I never purge. I was being maintained on the Olanzapine 2.5 mg for eleven years. I read a story of a woman who had a first psychotic break, and after she became lucid, she went off her medication, and her psychiatrist instructed her to go back on if she felt things getting weird. The premise would be that early on a person can have some insight. I have a feeling that since I was once on 15 mg and have now been on 2.5 mg for basically eleven years, I am safe. I stopped taking it months ago, and if necessary, will take it again. (I am not endorsing that anyone stop their psychotropic medications. This is always a discussion to have with the prescribing specialist). As part of my mental health hygiene, I know my limits and pace myself. Calvin called it my "anti-spiritual awakening drug" because someone once called my psychosis a spiritual awakening. Sometimes to be a turd, he accuses me of thinking in Comic Sans and/or crayon. I give it back to Calvin. I tell him he and the cat should start advertising their 'sleeping master class'. He also says he wants to lose weight but keeps eating four packs of noodles daily, so Amber made a picture that hangs in the front room that reads "Noodle House Diet Centre." Calvin gives me a hard time about my backing the car up, and how much better he is. I tell him I can't do better because I had psychosis. Best nonsensical excuse ever.

I accept fully that I have a severe mental illness, and I am actually thankful that I experienced it. That is not to say I want another psychotic break. I only say that because it has helped me finally develop the self-esteem and happiness that I wanted all my life. I am also uniquely situated to help my children should they become ill. Although I still care about my appearance, I don't lean on that for my self-esteem. I also learned sexual conquests have nothing to do with self-esteem. I am still uncomfortable with the idea of watching sci-fi things.

I love the life I have created. There are obvious risks with massage, but there are people in this world whose passions and abilities take them to dangerous jobs. Jobs that come to mind are volcanologists, rock climbers, cops, our front line healthcare professionals, and military personnel. Risk with hobbies and vocation is on a continuum. We take the precautions we can. In this way, we mitigate risk and are not sacrificing a higher value for a lower value. I am not going against my grain with massage. That said, I still want to help people. I have the tools, the drive, and the passion to make a difference.

I have been prescribed Breo for treatment of asthma for some years now. I no longer smoke. I started meditating on my lungs. My meditation for my lungs was always one of "breathing in love." There is an incredible little children's book called *The Samurai's Gift* written by Kristi Shimada, which is of value to any child or adult with asthma. I would encourage you to read this. If you are on any medication, do not stop taking it unless advised by your doctor.

I will offer an update on my children. Mingus is happy. He is a gamehead. I caught him singing yesterday :) He treats the cat like a dog, and it is so cute and funny. Tonight he accidentally spilled ginger ale on her. He tells me I should not use the word cute "against him," so I am biting my tongue all the time. He is a solid ten on a headstrong scale and loves gravy now. I love to rate everything from physical pain to you-name-it on a 1-10 scale. Sometimes I switch to percentage, for fun. Calvin jokes that Mingus thinks loud equals funny. Our neighbours put up a privacy fence, but we call it a sound barrier. I like to tease Mingus and Amber about their game music which, to me, sounds manic with no bass. I once purchased a JL Fathom Dual 12-inch and an entire stereo system with good towers, etc., set in motion by wanting to hear one song, *Love You Inside Out* by the Bee Gees, because it sounded so good on headphones. I experimented with the just-noticeable difference and habituation as an unwanted consequence. It was a bit crazy-making. There was concern about inadequate wiring in the house, worry about Lilly, timing the bus arrival, accessing it from Calvin's room, almost killing the song *September by* Earth Wind & Fire, keeping the neighbours off my back, and running around checking my precious ornaments.

I depend on Snoop Dog for some great humor content and to mention songs, including his own, new or old, when I have time to visit his Instagram. I enjoy Van Halen, The Cult, Kim Mitchell, Streetheart, George Michael and too many songs to name. My playlist is quite tired. Music will sometimes give me chills, like when Chaka Khan screams in *I Feel for You.* I must mention the most beautiful piece I know. I remember dancing to *Air* by Bach with Calvin in my arms when he was about two. I almost never cry, but it moves me to tears and suspends my ability to use a pen, if I have not listened to it for a while.

Amber is on fire with her art skills. I love beautiful color compositions, but for my entire life I cannot put color on paper and get any *wow* effect. Amber uses color in a way that I can't put into words. A recent piece she did feels addicting to me. I look at it frequently and linger over it. I would love to share her work but I am writing under a pen name for the twin's privacy.

Amber can keep up with her gaming brothers. I get schooled on gaming jargon. One day, I overheard one of them talking about a "bone welder". I had to check my hearing. When I asked what exactly that was, I was told it is a crafting tool. An ambitious term from the game world is 'grinding'. According to Amber, it means leveling up to become stronger. This term may have appeal when I apply it to messages for her own growth. I want to nurture her to feel pride in herself. What we want to avoid is "camping", which refers to players who stay in one place instead of actually playing the game. The application for personal growth is obvious.

Amber and I are on the same page for humor and I share Gary Larson's comics with her. I have to mention a couple or three or more favorites: *People Who Drove Too Slow in the Fast Lane Going to a Special Room in Hell, Scientist Hell: Psychics, Astrologists & Mediums Eternal Discussion, Alligator/Crocodile Quandary, Helen and I went to Hell and Back Vacation Picture with the Devil, Trick Spoon, Move Over and Let Me Drive on the Moon,* and *Professor Schnabel's Cleaning Lady Mistakes His Time Machine for a New Dryer.* I have a group chat with Amber and Calvin where I share funny Facebook memes, and there are many. Amber was joking with Calvin about the smoke detector malfunctioning and showing a green light. Calvin said, "green means Go, get out of the house!". So Amber started talking about red check marks and green x's and I instantly remembered "opposite days". One of the funniest things is when Calvin has Amber laughing so hard she is paralyzed on the floor. In all of this, I am trying to give my children the best chance at happiness and will be there for them if they experience mental illness.

I am not sure how this will hit, as family jokes have the context of understanding the personalities involved. Calvin was scanning and cataloging pictures of my dad from WW2. There were a number of pictures where my dad was smiling brightly. There was nothing in his character that would suggest anything sinister, and he valued life and respected others. He had a good character. He had never travelled before the war. Calvin, Amber, and Mingus' 'Grampie' served the country.

Faced with WW2, he somehow found happiness in that extreme, tragic, and uncertain environment. It looked to us like he was experimenting with hairstyles and growing a moustache, at one point. He was pictured smiling with one of his friends from the war, leaning inside what looked like a D-Day landing craft. There was a photo of him standing with some other guys in front of a downed German plane, or "Jerry kite", as he referred to it. There was a beach shot with war wreckage in the background, and his friend was smiling on a mound of sand. On the back of one photo, where he was in a dugout, he had written, "My own personal retreat". We started joking about so many smiling pictures, and called it "Grampie's epic war vacation" or "Grampie's relaxing vacation to Nazi-occupied France".

You might not be surprised Calvin has nothing to do with James, but he never speaks poorly about him in front of Amber and Mingus. Teenagers are naturally edgy, so he came up with a prank idea for James. The prank was to put up posters locally at grocery stores, telephone poles, and community boards. The posters would be styled like a "lost pet" notice picturing James with instructions "if found" to "call James" (on his own number). It hasn't happened, but it would be funny.

There was one other funny thing Calvin did. I accidentally sent a red heart to James by text when I meant to send a smile emoji following some details for Amber and Mingus. I told Calvin of the mistake, and he immediately got five friends to spam James with red hearts. I was holding my head laughing and sweating at the same time.

James falls down on some communication with me by spells, but I know he loves Mingus and Amber with all his heart. Since I never like to pass up a chance to share a laugh, I had to share the following with James. One day I received a call from a doctor's office asking if she could speak with Mingus. I said, "I am his mom so you can talk to me." She then said that Mingus was scheduled for hemorrhoid surgery in another week. I asked her if she was sure, and she said, "Yes." I asked her when Mingus had the initial consultation, and she said, "Three months ago." I was thinking to myself, "Holy Cats, I know James doesn't tell me much, but this is crazy!!!" I questioned her again saying that Mingus was only eleven years old, I knew nothing about it, and it seemed strange. She then realized Mingus had been mixed up with a forty-year-old patient. It was too funny not to share, and James took the poke and had a laugh at his own expense.

Calvin loves table salt—he might even like road salt—and he has determined we have 'fast' and 'slow' salt shakers. He has a salt shaker in his bedroom. When I ask him if he wants something to eat, he asks if it is salty food. From my horse days, I am imagining the perfect Christmas gift for him: a salt lick. The large size is about 40 lbs; there is also a mineralized version. We have seen mountain goats on BBC Earth take dizzying risks for salt, but I feel like Calvin might be missing the whole point of eating.

I want to share another ongoing fun activity between us. I started rescuing spiders in the house and taking them outside. We have special spider "rescue boxes". Amber loves it, and we have "briefings" on spider-related activity. I can never get over the fact that they actually perceive the exact moment I see them. I know this because they freeze. Are they watching my eyes or the orientation of my body? We say we are building up credit with the universe. Ironically or unironically, we have had some significant good things happen directly following spider rescues. For example, James was agreeable on a critical health care issue which flabbergasted me. When these good things happened, we became more invested in the spider rescues. One day, I accidentally vacuumed a spider, and Calvin wanted to make sure it was not intentional. He warned me we might need to start building a bomb shelter under the house if it had not been accidental. Having fun, we tied a completely unrelated mystery into the spider narrative. Somehow, I had been added to a mailing list on the other side of the planet. It was an Australian major retailer, and I could not remove myself or block it. It comes every Monday without fail. We concluded the spiders from Australia were trying to reach us to get us to do rescues there. We know Australia has hand-sized spiders that actually hiss, so that means spiders with more personality. I heard there are some speed runner spiders there that can outrun a man and are seriously weaponized. They seem like they might need to calm down. It makes me wonder what mission they are solving on the evolutionary to-do list. I'd like to imagine they are protecting the beautiful opals.

A little update on Lilly, who the children say is also a Zoomer. Lilly recently had to go to the vet. She needed blood work, and when they took her to another room to have her neck shaved for the blood draw, I heard them say, "She is strong!" Calvin has been laughing and saying that Lilly fought "two vets." Really it was two assistants, but it sounds better saying "two vets." She ended up on the most expensive vet food possible, which leaves me with the feeling we are actually leasing her from the vet. Lee says Lilly is "over talkative," which is a bit true. She keeps track of every family member and howls at the bottom of the stairs when someone goes upstairs. Sweet girl.

I will give an honorable mention to our '99 Tercel. Princess Tercel has been dependable and safely transported Calvin, Amber, Mingus, Lilly, and myself for many years. The dynamics of guitar and bass, full-on with the sub, in Bryan Adam's *Cuts Like a Knife* in the car is crazy good. I have had more than a couple people urge me in the direction of updating my car. I reply with, "Do you sell family members?" The children back me up. I was at a gas station one day, and a tow truck driver was close to me as I was getting in the car. I jokingly said to him, "You aren't getting this!" He seemed to be on a sleepwalking frequency, and when he started to come to he said, "Yeah?" We have rescued a bird and a turtle in the car. I have a critter-catching container in the trunk in case we find something. When Calvin, Lee, and I were in California, we went to an exotic car dealership. I was offered a ride in a Ferrari and was drooling, but I wanted Calvin to have the experience. The salesman asked me what I was driving, and I answered honestly and dignified his time by commenting that I just loved cars, which I knew he would understand. Calvin is looking to buy his first car. He laughed at the search results for his price range with cars in backyards with their tires "melted into the ground".

I found myself in the middle of a property dispute involving usage rights for the driveway at the seaside insane asylum yesterday. There is a dedicated Facebook page for the community. I almost don't dare mention there are rental opportunities there if you know the right person. Mingus recently shared a funny meme with me that said, "I bought the whole speedometer so I am going to use the whole speedometer". I related it to my current crisis and I thought to myself, "If I am being forced to spend money on litigation, I am going to enjoy it like a vacation". Homer said to me, "It is the fun of making money that makes money", so I was thinking it could be the fun of going to court that could help me win, but I will make peace with any outcome. I am book-poor currently, so I was thinking about money for the process. I had a fun idea that I will not act on because it would be abrasive, but it keeps me in good spirits. I imagined I could post on the Facebook page the following for the "Storybook people": "Betting opportunity: a 50/50 draw to raise capital for a squatting rights squabble. The property dispute winner takes 50%. Then I had the entertaining thought that I was going to keep going until I found a judge who agrees with me. I primed my lawyer by telling her we were going to think of the property line as a 'rough estimate'. Angelina laughed when I told her. As her incredible nature affords, she will not ruffle any feathers and remains on good terms with my neighbour and myself simultaneously. She can get around the most sensitive situations with ease and grace that is mind-boggling. Angelina has a covert strength and open mind that catches me off guard at times. Perhaps a slight appetite for risk, methinks. Calvin says everyone needs an Angelina in their life.

I was discussing it with Calvin, and we agreed that judges must get weary of the frequent use of the victim card in these kinds of matters. (I also reminded Calvin the last time I went down to the cottage alone I had a text from him asking me how to turn off the fire alarm at home.) We are going to cook a fun story and invite my 'tiger' lawyer to enjoy herself, too. I know it is easy to think, 'She will, taking your money to the bank'. I don't begrudge her success, earnings, or brains. She should enjoy any fun coming her way.

In an exhausted state today from lots of late edits and a deadline to launch, I need to find another focus to keep my mind occupied or go to sleep to stop the creative inspiration. In that state, Calvin was driving us to the grocery store. He was forgetting to close the garage door, so I said, "Close the drawer", then corrected myself to say, "…As we drive out of the kitchen". Then he stopped at the mailbox and was poky, so I said, "Hurry up or the book will get longer". I feel like I don't have enough time to pick out clothes, and what I do wear feels more like a uniform.

My mom wanted me in a neat package, but, perhaps admitting defeat, she once said I was a free spirit. I wish her and my dad eternal joy… My children, all the happiness, self-esteem, and laughter they can stand. I am fifty-two years old and it took me a long time to get to this place. My wish for everyone else is to achieve high self-esteem and happiness faster than I did—that is my purpose.

I want to say to the voyeurs, "You're welcome". Curiosity, if it is not intrusive, seems PC. I read tabloids, and they push the boundaries of intrusiveness. I am unlikely to stop enjoying them. I am also fascinated by albinism and follow someone on social media for that reason. Lee has said there will be another book, and two are possible. I have one which will have more important information about insight and intention that is begging for my attention. If there was a third book, it would be a celebration compilation of funny psychosis stories from people who have made peace with mental illness, are healed, and can find humor. Although, in my experience, mental illness hides incredible pain, I believe humans can hold two realities in their mind at one time. Gary Larson captured this in his comic where a patient was perched on the top of a coat hanger. The patient was wearing two party hats, a life preserver, and flippers. The therapist said, "So, Mr Fenton...let's begin with your mother".

Mental illness sufferers of the world... unite.

CONCLUSION

"We must recognise the possibility of change and believe in the self we are now in the process of becoming. That old sense of self and failure must go. It is false, and we are not to believe what is false."
—*Maltz*

A fun self-help book... she said. Being happy, laughing, and feeling high self-esteem is fun and I want that for you. Self-discovery with the tools to achieve this is exciting. There is no ceiling on feeling good. We just need to remove the lid and have some high octane strategies. Anemic thinking didn't work. One of Shakespeare's characters said, "Nothing was good or bad but only that thinking made it so." Shakespeare needed Homer for the "how to" part (grin). This puzzle of how to achieve happiness and high self-esteem is complete. You can see the depth of psychiatric problems I had and was helped. The first issue I wanted you to explore was happiness anxiety. It is wasted effort to attempt feeling better if you have an unwritten script that says happiness is somehow wrong for you. You do have a right to be happy no matter what early learning might have taught you and no matter what you have gone through recently. I want you out of pain. You can be very far down and start praising yourself straight away. Today! It is a gentleness applied to yourself based on the idea that thinking and behavior improve when we feel better.

See yourself as that confident woman or man who is buoyant and able to face anything. When you realize many things are just *wants* and not *needs*, you will relax. This relaxation will make you more vibrant to be around for your children, romantic partner, and friends. As you cast off your self-criticism and worry habits that make you experience self-pity and depression, you will have more energy to pursue your goals and interests. You will be a one punch knockout. Don't label pain as being smart... tell the truth. Stretch to become comfortable with praising yourself. Remember, you cannot have too much pride. Don't let anyone tell you otherwise. *Your self-esteem will be a brick house instead of a straw one.*

The more you commit and experiment with these techniques, the more you will experience the benefits. I challenge you to start with 3% effort. Anyone can do 3%. It is a place to start and will be easy for you. Commit and hit send. You can be happy and have high self-esteem. You are amazing as you are. The mirror works perfectly!

My closing remarks are this: One of the best secrets of the universe is this: *Playfulness* and *intention* to do good toward yourself and others. With your self-esteem secured and never on the line, you will not be as concerned about outcomes, win or lose. I want to be in step with what God would want from me, in my everyday life and in helping others.

If you implement these ideas, please rate your projected score:
Your level of happiness 1–10
Your level of self-esteem 1–10

GG
xo

Laura Midna
"Setting the world on fire one person at a time"

ABOUT THE AUTHOR

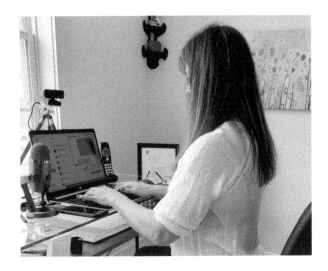

Laura Midna is a life coach with extensive personal and professional knowledge of the suffering that accompanies mental illness. She is passionate about offering the best practices available to achieve high self-esteem, happiness, and romantic success. Her confidence comes from successfully answering the question, "How can I feel amazing despite my severe mental illness history?" Laura is currently living with her three children and pet cat. Her goal is to inspire anyone who wants to settle the issue of self-esteem and happiness once and for all.

Can You Help?

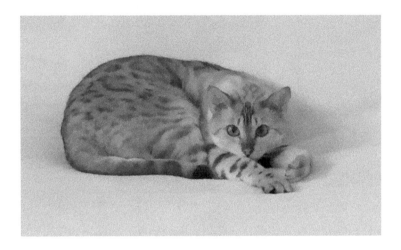

Thank you so much for reading my book! Please post an honest review of what you thought of the book on your favourite online retailer. This helps me achieve a better virtual bookshelf in stores and aids in discoverability of the book for people who may benefit from my brand of help. If you are in a positive recovery position and want to contribute funny psychosis stories, please reach out.

Thanks so much,
Laura Midna

If you want individual support, I've included my contact information.

Email:
lauramidna1969@gmail.com

Website:
https://lauramidna.wixsite.com/lauramidna

Social Media:
https://twitter.com/laura_midna

https://www.linkedin.com/in/laura-midna-7772121b7

https://www.facebook.com/Laura-Midna-108752564274737

https://instagram.com/lauramidna

REFERENCE LIST

Adyashanti. (2016, Nov. 9). *"There is only one thing..."* Twitter. URL. https://twitter.com/Adyashanti/status/796425173272399872?s=20

Bowen, M. (2020). *Surviving the unthinkable.* Markus Pierre Bowen Jr.

Branden, N. (1994). *The six pillars of self-esteem.* New York, N.Y.: Bantam.

Branden, N. (1998) Series of three in-person interviews at his home in Beverly Hills and 7-10 interviews over the phone.

Carnegie, D. (1981). *How to win friends and influence people.* New York: Simon & Schuster Inc.

Francetić, R. (2020). *The power of human energy.* Renata Francetić.

Gallagher, S. (2018). *Understanding the fear of success.* Proctor Gallagher Institute. https://www.proctorgallagherinstitute.com/383401/understanding-the-fear-of-success?fbclid=lWAR1okrT6gimax9bYFaRddTsok8cuBNyT97XAU86Q:1S0rwn9DkWgnOeH

Hayden, A. (2018). *Does visualization work? The shocking truth about the law of attraction.* https://redpilltheory.com/2018/07/01/does-visualization-work-the-uncensored-truth-about-the-law-of-attraction/

Henley, D. (1982). "Dirty laundry." *I Can't Stand Still.* Universal Production Music.

Jakes, T.D. (2014, Nov. 5). *Steps Video for Thought T D Jakes.* Sha Jan.

Katie, B. (2011). *Loving what is.* New York: Random House USA Inc.

Larson, G. (2003). *The complete farside.* Kansas City, Mo: Andrews McMeel Pub.

Maltz, M. (2015). *Psycho-cybernetics.* New York, New York: Perigee An Imprint of Penguin Random House LLC.

McDonald, H. (2010). *Advanced sessions.* Winter Haven, Florida: NewInformation!, Inc.

McDonald, H. (2007-2016). Estimating 25 personal interviews by phone.

McDonald, H. (1999-2006). *Stop your divorce.* Winter Haven, Florida: NewInformation!, Inc.

Miller, G. (2016, Oct. 26). *Pimp my wheelchair.* TVFilthyFrank. https://youtu.be/bkdeqeP7VUO

National Institute of Mental Health. (2020). *What is psychosis.* https://www.nimh.nih.gov

Peele, S. (1999). *The diseasing of America.* San Francisco, California: Lexington/Jossey-Bass.

Placeboing. (2017, June 22). *Gay frogs.* Alex Jones REMIX. https://youtu.be/9JRLCBb7qK8

Poni, J. (2020). *Follow your curiosity.* Joe Poni.

Proctor, B. (2015). *You were born rich.* Scottsdale, Arizona: Proctor Gallagher Institute.

Remondino, G. (2020). *Genius by choice.* Giulia Remondino.

Robbins, T. (2018, April 6). *How to create an a-ha moment.* https://youtu.be/24ooUBw7mko

Rowell, M. (2021). *Leadership upgrade.* Michael Rowell.

Shimada, K. (2020). *The Samurai's gift.* Kristi Shimada.

Reference List

Winfrey, O, & Chopra, D. (2016, Feb. 22). *Deepak Chopra showed Oprah the power of her mind.* https://youtu.be/bAbQUO9x_8g

Yates, M. (2020). *Happy, joyous, and free.* Melanie Yates.

My formatter, Jen Henderson, did formatting acrobatics for me. It is difficult to turn off the creative tap just because it is time. To all the formatters who format books 'one sentence at a time', this is for you!

Lightning Source UK Ltd.
Milton Keynes UK
UKHW012201210921
390987UK00001B/23